Assisted Reproductive Technologies in the Global South and North

Assisted Reproductive Technologies in the Global South and North critically analyses the political and social frameworks of Assisted Reproductive Technology (ART), and its impact in different countries. In the context of a worldwide social pressure to conceive – particularly for women – this collection explores the effect of the development of ARTs, growing globalisation and reproductive medicalisation on global societies.

Providing an overview of the issues surrounding ART, both in the Global South and North, this book analyses ART inequalities, commonalities and specificities in various countries, regions and on the transnational scene. From a multidisciplinary perspective and drawing on multisite studies, it highlights some new issues relating to ART (e.g. egg freezing, surrogacy) and discusses some older issues regarding infertility and its medical treatment (e.g. in vitro fertilisation, childless stigmatisation and access to treatment).

This book aims to redress the balance between what is known about Assisted Reproductive Technologies in the Global North, and how the issue is investigated in the Global South. It aims to draw out the global similarities in the challenges that ARTs bring between these different areas of the world. It will appeal to scholars and students in the social sciences, medicine, public health, health policy, women's and gender studies and demography.

Virginie Rozée is a researcher in sociology at the French Institute for Demographic Studies (INED), France. She is working on gender and reproductive health and rights issues (abortion, contraception, infertility, assisted reproductive technologies, cross-border reproductive care, surrogacy) in different geographical areas (Europe, Latin America, India).

Sayeed Unisa is a professor at the International Institute for Population Sciences (IIPS), India. Her research interests are gender issues, infertility, and nutrition. She has done a longitudinal study of infertile couples from Andhra Pradesh, India. She has received the Royan International award for her research work on infertility. She was also involved in a project on 'prevention and management of infertility in India'.

Routledge Studies in the Sociology of Health and Illness

Assisted Reproductive Technologies in the Global South and North

Issues, challenges and the future

Edited by Virginie Rozée and Sayeed Unisa

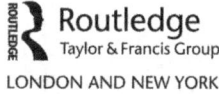

LONDON AND NEW YORK

First published 2016
by Routledge
2 Park Square, Milton Park, Abingdon, Oxon OX14 4RN

and by Routledge
711 Third Avenue, New York, NY 10017

Routledge is an imprint of the Taylor & Francis Group, an informa business

First issued in paperback 2022

British Library Cataloguing-in-Publication Data
A catalogue record for this book is available from the British Library

Library of Congress Cataloging-in-Publication Data
Names: Rozée Gomez, Virginie, editor. | Unisa, Sayeed, editor.
Title: Assisted reproductive technologies in the global south and north : issues, challenges and the future / edited by Virginie Rozâee Gomez and Sayeed Unisa.
Description: Milton Park, Abingdon, Oxon ; New York, NY : Routledge, 2016. |
Series: Routledge studies in the sociology of health and illness Identifiers: LCCN 2016002027 | ISBN 9781138932357 (hardback) | ISBN 9781315679310 (e-book)
Subjects: LCSH: Human reproductive technology.
Classification: LCC RG133.5 .A86 2016 | DDC 618.1/7806--dc23
LC record available at http://lccn.loc.gov/2016002027

ISBN: 978-1-138-93235-7 (hbk)
ISBN: 978-0-367-22402-8 (pbk)
ISBN: 978-1-315-67931-0 (ebk)

Typeset in Times New Roman
by Saxon Graphics Ltd, Derby

Contents

Contributors

BENABED Aïcha, University of Oran, Algeria

BIRENBAUM-CARMELI Daphna, University of Haifa, Israel

CORRÊA Marilena, State University of Rio de Janeiro (UERJ), Brazil

DUCHESNE Véronique, Université Paris Descartes, Sorbonne Paris Cité, France

HVIDTFELDT Karen, University of Southern Denmark, Denmark

LANCE Delphine, École des Hautes Études en Sciences Sociales (EHESS), France

MARWAH Vrinda, SAMA: Resource Group for Women and Health, India

MERCHANT Jennifer, University Paris 2 Panthéon-Assas, France

NADIMPALLY Sarojini, SAMA: Resource Group for Women and Health, India

NAGARAJAN Nagadeepti, Gynaecworld: The Center for Women's Health and Fertility, India

PUJARI Sucharita, National Institute of Rural Development and Panchayati Raj (NIRDPR), India

RASOOL Sabahat, Gynaecworld: The Center for Women's Health and Fertility, India

ROZÉE Virginie, French Institute for Demographic Studies, France

RUDRAPPA Sharmila, University of Texas, United States

SHAH Duru, Gynaecworld: The Center for Women's Health and Fertility, India

SHENFIELD Françoise, University College London Hospitals, United Kingdom

TEMAN Elly, Ruppin Academic Center, Israel

UNISA Sayeed, International Institute for Population Sciences, India

WHITTAKER Andrea, Monash University, Australia

ZEGERS-HOCHSCHILD Fernando, University Diego Portales, Chile

Foreword

Assisted Reproductive Technologies are re-shaping the traditional understanding of reproduction and motherhood. Operating within a profoundly gendered context, these new technologies are opening up new discourses and conflicts based on the ways in which they impact women, and reinforce the notions of family, gender identities and reproductive rights.

United Nations Population Fund (UNFPA) has been engaging with the discourse on ARTs to understand the implications of ART for women's reproductive health and rights. Since 2010, UNFPA has supported evidence generation and creation of a knowledge base on the complexities surrounding ARTs and commercial surrogacy to guide policy dialogue and advocacy in India.

It is in this context that in October 2014, UNFPA collaborated with the Institut National d'Etudes Démographiques (INED, Paris, France), the International Institute for Population Sciences (IIPS), and the Centre de Population et de Développement (CEPED, Paris, France) to organize an international seminar on 'Assisted Reproductive Technologies in Northern and Southern Countries: Issues, Challenges & the Future'. The seminar aimed to provide a critical view of ARTs from different country contexts and approaches, and to build understanding on the implications, concerns, challenges and response mechanisms related to ARTs, across borders. The idea for a publication based on the papers presented at the conference, documenting the different perspectives and experiences with ARTs thus took shape.

This publication offers an overview of ART techniques and regulatory mechanisms in different countries alongwith the associated implications and concerns. The countries included in the review, are represented by their regional presence- Global South (Brazil, India, Thailand, Australia and Africa) and Global North (France, Israel, United-Kingdom, and Europe). The experience of ART across different countries serves to highlight the central role played by ART in medical tourism in an expanding global market as those seeking ART services travel to countries where ART is relatively more affordable or where the modalities are more flexible.

The book also aims to shed light on (un)common controversies and challenges regarding medical issues, ethical concerns, and commercial practices, around reproduction. For instance, ARTs are hailed by some especially in the context of the stigma associated with childlessness. On the other hand, it is argued that the availability of ARTs may further reinforce the social pressure on women to bear a child. Furthermore there is growing concern that the development of ARTs in the midst of increasing reproductive medicalization and commercialization may deepen inequalities between those who can afford such treatments and those who can't, between clients of ART services and those who offer their reproductive capacities-often times women who are poor or vulnerable. The publication emphasizes the need for further research and deeper investigation on ART and commercial surrogacy particularly in low-resource countries and in the transnational scenario.

The perspectives related to new reproductive technologies may be debatable, but at the centre of these perspectives are the rights of women. It is in this spirit that UNFPA welcomes this publication to foster sharing and exchange of multiple perspectives and insights for a more informed policy discourse on ARTs.

This book will be interesting reading for policy makers who are confronted with the question of instituting or administering regulation on ARTs and commercial surrogacy and practitioners working on these issues. This book will also be useful for experts to learn from the legal and policy environment around ARTs and commercial surrogacy across countries.

I would like to congratulate the editors for making this compilation possible, and appreciation must be accorded to the contributors for their wide and diverse coverage of the different aspects of ARTs.

Diego Palacios
UNFPA Representative for India &
Country Director for Bhutan

Acknowledgements

This book is the result of a fruitful collaboration between us. Thanks to the Marie Curie Programme of European Commission, it has given us the opportunity to work together since 2013 on surrogacy issues in India through the Research project called "Micro-realities of surrogacy in India" (Surrog-India).

The plan for the book took shape through the discussion on Assisted Reproductive Technologies we engaged in during an international seminar organized by us in Mumbai, India, in 2014. This event was supported by the National Institute for Demographic Studies (INED, Paris, France), International Institute for Population Sciences (IIPS, Mumbai, India), United Nations Population Fund (UNFPA, Delhi, India) and Centre de Population et de Development (CEPED, Paris, France) and we sincerely thank these institutions. This seminar gave us the opportunity to exchange on ART issues in different countries and regions. Different societies face specific challenges related to their historical, political, economic and social backgrounds; but also common challenges with the growing globalization, the progressive transformations of kinship and parenthood, and the increasing reproductive medicine advances. This seminar also highlighted that ART issues, especially in southern countries and on the transnational scene, existed and some techniques and practices were undocumented. That encouraged us to suggest and then edit a timely book, trying to represent the diversity of the situations with relevant analysis.

We would like to thank all the contributors for their key work they accepted to share, for their positive disposition and support in reviewing and updating their chapters along with their usual work.

We would like to express our sincere gratitude to the institutions and persons who supported, morally and financially, our initiative and all of those who helped and assisted us in this collective adventure.

We are deeply grateful to Routledge Publishing House for its trust, enthusiasm, and efficiency in handling the planning and production of this book.

Virginie Rozée and Sayeed Unisa

Introduction

Virginie Rozée & Sayeed Unisa

Infertility is a prevalent reproductive health problem. It is estimated that 80 million people worldwide are infertile, i.e. between 4 to 14 percent of people (Nachtigall, 2006). Since the 1980s, advances in medicine have made it possible to overcome the problems of infertility through assisted reproductive technology (ART). However, "at the dawn of the twenty-first century, assisted reproduction continues to be a source of ambivalence" (Storrow, 2006). ART makes it possible to fulfil the desire for a child regardless of infertility problems, marital situation, age or sexual orientation. At the same time, use of ART may reinforce existing inequalities, and it questions ethical principles and traditional values.

More controversies arose when progress made possible the use of donors (for sperm, oocyte or embryo donation) and surrogates to assist reproduction. These debates concern the medicalisation of healthy bodies, the possible exploitation of women who offer their reproductive capacities, the creation of new families and the dissociation of the reproductive process. Surrogacy and oocyte donation are particularly controversial in terms of their medical and sociological impacts, especially when they take place in "less developed countries" (Sen, 1990). This is particularly true of surrogacy in India, which has become a contentious "mother destination" (Rudrappa, 2010).

Infertility care and use of ART is well documented in the Global North countries, including Australia. Nevertheless, few researchers have covered the issue of infertility and use of ART in less developed countries (mainly situated in the Global South). Little is known about infertility, related palliative care and childlessness in Southern countries, which mainly target family planning and population growth control. However, infertility and ART in the Global South is a real health and social issue. Little is also known of Eastern countries, with low resources, that are generally considered to practise cheap but unethical ART (although there are no empirical data to support this view).

The objective of the present book is to analyse ART inequalities, commonalities and specificities in various parts of the world. It offers a critical analysis of the political, medical, cultural and social frameworks of ART and its impacts in different countries and regions from the Global South (Algeria, Brazil, India, Thailand) and Eastern countries such as Ukraine, as well as the Global North (Israel, United Kingdom, United States) and Australia. India receives particular attention here as a perfect illustration of ART issues worldwide, with the rapid growth of its "ART industry" (SAMA Team, 2007) in an unregulated context. India is often described in international media as a risky destination for ART.

The book brings together multidisciplinary and multisite studies and explores various fields of ART. Its chapters present various perspectives from the disciplines of anthropology, demography, medicine, law, sociology and public health, covering different countries and diverse populations. Various ART techniques, namely in vitro fertilisation, egg donation, egg freezing and surrogacy, are also covered. Different issues are approached: legal and medical regulations governing infertility and ART; social, cultural and religious representations; and the medical and personal experiences of those involved, on both the local and transnational scenes.

Existing studies point out that further in-depth research is needed on ART and its management and impacts on the transnational scene (Inhorn and Gürtin, 2011). This book contributes to improving knowledge and understanding of transnational ART. ART has become a burning issue and the subject of controversies and debates regarding medical issues, ethical concerns, commercial practices and "convenience" (social) uses. Providing new empirical and analytical elements, this book sheds light on these debates and controversies. It offers an extensive overview of the contemporary context of ART and its issues, and distances itself from a monolithic perspective to create a wider understanding of both common and particular aspects of ART around the world.

Infertility and concepts and issues in ART

Assisted reproductive technologies cannot be investigated without first exploring the issue of infertility, the magnitude of this health and social concern and its context and representation. According to the World Health Organization (WHO), infertility is defined as a failure to obtain pregnancy after 12 months or more of regular unprotected sexual intercourse (Zegers-Hochschild et al., 2009). The global infertility problem could be due to late marriage, postponement of pregnancy, high prevalence of sexually transmitted infections and other infections or consequences of childbirth or abortion in unsafe sanitary conditions (Nachtigall, 2006). Some researchers have also pointed out that pollution and pesticides may be responsible for infertility. Infertility is particularly prevalent in less developed countries. Marcia Inhorn reported that according to a global study based on 47 demographic and health surveys in low-resource countries, more than 186 million married women of reproductive age (15–49 years) were infertile (Inhorn, 2009). In her chapter on African experiences, Véronique Duchesne speaks of an "infertility belt" identified in the sub-Saharan region: there, in countries like Zimbabwe, 30% of couples may suffer secondary infertility (Nachtigall, 2006).

Infertility has a cultural and social impact on the life of couples, especially on women. In his chapter that draws a portrait of infertility in the world, particularly in Latin America, Fernando Zegers-Hochschild argues that infertility has the same effects as coronary disease, cancer or HIV. Infertility is stigmatising all over the world, especially for women. In the majority of countries, women are socially expected to become mothers and to ensure the descendance of the family. There is, therefore, a social pressure on women to conceive (Inhorn and van Balen, 2002; Donchin, 2010). If pregnancy is delayed or never occurs, then women are considered as responsible for this failure. Sarojini Nadimpally and Vrinda Marwah in their chapter analyse the gender impacts of infertility and ART in India. The authors describe the discrimination against women in infertile couples. The infertile female body is considered by society as a non-performing body, as a perverted and polluted body, and the woman is considered as not sufficiently devoted to her husband. They explain that "the personal imaginary of infertility seems disproportionately affected by gender" and women even lose respect in society. Indeed, in India as in many other countries, infertility has several negative impacts. It may lead to stigmatised marital instability, emotional harassment and low self-esteem (Jejeebhoy, 1998; Unisa, 1999). In Algeria, Aicha Benabed comes to similar conclusions from an anthropological perspective based on interviews with women who underwent ART. In some other African countries, Véronique Duchesne explains that infertility is associated with women's vulnerability to witchcraft.

Men in infertile couples are less subject to stigmatisation and discrimination. Male infertility is still socially unknown or taboo and is protected by the wife, who, if her husband is infertile, does not reveal the fact (Rozée and Mazuy, 2012). Except for the anthropological works of Marcia Inhorn in Lebanon and Egypt (Inhorn, 2004), the male experience of infertility (whatever the medical problem or its origin) is poorly studied in the scientific literature. The chapter by Sucharita Pujari and Sayeed Unisa is very relevant as it investigates men's perspectives and experiences of infertility among childless married men in the Indian state of Andhra Pradesh. The authors reported that men are often ignorant and do not realise that they too could be responsible for the inability to have a child. Most of them consider that the woman is primarily responsible for children.

There are two main techniques in ART: artificial insemination (AI) and in vitro fertilisation (IVF). In AI, sperm is introduced in utero (i.e. in the woman's body) to help with in vivo fertilisation. AI can be performed with sperm from the woman's partner or a donor (who may or may not be anonymous). Depending on the reports and research, AI is not always considered as part of ART. In IVF, fertilisation takes place in vitro, i.e. outside the woman's body, in a test tube (which is why babies born from this technique are commonly called "test-tube babies"). IVF can be performed with the intended parents' gametes (sperm, oocytes) and/or with gametes from donors (egg donor, sperm donor) or through embryo donation (Zegers-Hochschild et al., 2009). The embryo is then transferred to the mother's uterus or the uterus of a surrogate. The woman who receives the embryo and carries the future baby until birth for another woman, man or couple is called a "surrogate" or "surrogate mother" and the person or persons for whom she is carrying the baby are known as the intended/intending/commissioning mother/father/parents.

Duru Shah, Sabahat Rasool and Nagadeepti Nagarajan in their chapter present a medical perspective and explain the history of surrogacy, particularly in India, its various uses and procedures. They also describe the various types of surrogacy practised in the world. The most common is gestational surrogacy, where the surrogate has not provided her own eggs. This book has a particular focus on surrogacy, as it is the most controversial medical ART practice in the world, mainly when it is transnational and involves a financial transaction between poor women from developing countries and couples from developed or rich countries.

In vitro fertilisation can be also performed with gametes that are frozen. A very new technology is known as egg/oocyte freezing or vitrification, depending on the technique used for freezing. It allows women to preserve fertility. However, it offers no guarantee that conception will take place and a baby will be delivered. This technique is now giving positive results (Dondorp et al., 2012; Cobo et al., 2013; Cobo et al., 2014). In the chapter by Daphna Birenbaum-Carmeli, this emergent and controversial technique of egg freezing is addressed with the example of Israel. Egg freezing gives hope to women with cancer that they will be able to conceive after their treatment (X-ray and chemotherapy seriously damage fertility), and it also allows women to conceive at a later age. There is, therefore, no consensus in the worldwide medical and political community regarding voluntary late motherhood. Beyond the ethical aspects, egg freezing also allows egg-banking for donation. In chapters by Françoise Shenfield and Marilena Corrêa, egg sharing between women who are undergoing IVF treatment and other women is reported to be prevalent in European countries and Brazil. It could therefore reduce the long waiting lists observed in some European countries (Pennings, 2004; Shenfield et al., 2011). On the other hand, there is hidden commercialisation in the practice of egg sharing in Brazil.

All the above-mentioned techniques which constitute ART are not possible, accessible or available worldwide for political, socio-cultural or financial reasons. This book highlights the diversity and the pluralism of ART regulation, practices and representations.

ART regulation, practices and access

Worldwide, there are particular inequalities in access to ART: many countries have no or very few specialised centres, do not offer ART facilities or do not accept such techniques at all. Regulation, practices and access vary from country to country (Rozée, 2011). Countries may have specific laws or general laws in the form of guidelines that are therefore not compulsory, or may rely on jurisprudence. Even within the same country (generally, a federal state), legal or political frameworks are diverse. ART regulations in certain countries prohibit or restrict some techniques and access to them. On the other hand, some encourage the use of ART, even for social reasons (as in Israel; see Birenbaum-Carmeli in this book). A given technique such as surrogacy may be available or practised differently in different countries. In the chapter by Andrea Whittaker, the rules and regulations of ART in Australia are described, while Delphine Lance and Jennifer Merchant present the scenario in the United States. In Australia, surrogacy is authorised in some states and prohibited in others. When surrogacy is permitted, it must be altruistic. Delphine Lance and Jennifer Merchant also show the piecemeal approach to surrogacy in the United States (see the map in their chapter).

Another strong disparity concerns state support and the ART sector (public vs private), which may condition the use of these techniques by a low-income population. While some countries offer state funding (as in France and Israel), the majority of countries provide no financial support for ART treatment. Generally, and mostly in less developed and emerging countries, infertility is not approached as a public health matter with specific public policies and possibly a social insurance system. In some countries, the main preoccupation is population growth and how to limit it (as in India and African countries); in others, the priority is to promote contraception and avoid unsafe abortion (in Latin America, as presented in this book by Zegers-Hochschild). Therefore, ART is generally unknown and disregarded in the general population, or seen as a "convenience". Fernando Zegers-Hochschild explains that not considering infertility as a public health matter like any other disorder may have dramatic consequences. It is estimated that in Latin America 14,000 couples suffer infertility problems. He states:

> One of the consequences of the absence of national regulatory bodies is that important decisions are left uncontrolled: the number of embryos to be transferred, the age limits for undergoing oocyte donation, anonymity of donors, economic compensation and access to treatment for same-sex couples and single women, among others.

Not being a public issue, ART has become a growing business and an unregulated market (Whittaker, 2011), even sometimes a black market where there is no law; the market is generally taken up by private providers and clinics for wealthy nationals and foreigners. All over the world, ART is in fact mainly performed in private centres. Marilena Corrêa states in her chapter that in Brazil, 90 percent of specialised centres are private. Hence, the access of ART services is a "matter of income or economic power". Because of the high cost, many nationals cannot afford such treatment. According to Fernando Zegers-Hochschild, this inequality in the access to fertility treatments violates the universal access to reproductive health promoted by the Millennium Development Goals (MDG). The book points out these inequalities in access to ART services within a same country in the chapters by Nadimpally and Marwah, Benabed, and Corrêa, and inequalities in cross-border reproductive care are addressed by Hvidtfeldt, Duchesne and Whittaker.

The diversity of regulations and possibilities has created a new social and medical phenomenon: cross-border reproductive care (CBRC) (Shenfield et al., 2010; Collins and Cook, 2010; Hudson et al., 2011; Rozée and de La Rochebrochard, 2013). CBRC is "a widespread phenomenon where infertile patients or collaborators (such as egg donors or potential surrogates) cross international borders in order to obtain or provide reproductive treatment outside their home country" (Shenfield et al., 2011). CBRC is considered as a worldwide and growing phenomenon (Ferraretti et al., 2010; Gürtin and Inhorn, 2011). It is the result of growing globalisation, network development and the increasing medicalisation of reproduction. ART, including transnational ART, is generally considered as a better option for infertile women, men and couples than another alternative such as adoption which is considered to be very limited and even more expensive.

CBRC transcends the context of origin and country of destination. Evidence suggests that CBRC is a matter of concern in the United Kingdom, which is considered to be one of the most flexible and open countries in Europe with regard to ART. Zeynep Gürtin and Marcia Inhorn (2011) put forward four main reasons why people and couples seek ART treatment in other countries: legal and religious prohibitions; financial considerations; quality and safety concerns; and personal preferences. Andrea Whittaker in her chapter analyses how and why such transnational use, in particular for surrogacy, has increased in Australia: about ten Australian children have been born through surrogacy within the country compared with some hundreds of babies through transnational surrogacy (i.e. performed in another country). While CBRC extends the field of possibilities to conceive a baby, it may create new problems and accentuate pre-existing inequalities (Storrow, 2010; Whittaker, 2011; Nahman, 2013).

The prohibition of some practices may have "perverse effects" and may displace the problem elsewhere, through CBRC. Reading through the chapters of this book, we learn that in the countries where ART has become a market or a reproductive industry, there is either an absence of legal regulations or insufficient regulations. This book stresses that ethical concerns are neglected and medical risks are higher where there is no regulation, but also that regulation can sometimes be useless or insufficient. ART may imply a liberal approach, governed by the ethics (and economic interests) of the physicians themselves. In the absence of regulations, the ART market can lead to hazardous practices, generally for the purposes of profit for clinics and agencies. ART patients may face risks: social and medical risks for egg donors or surrogates, legal problems for intended parents (Crozier and Martin, 2012).

The social and medical risks of ART are approached in several chapters. Sarojini Nadimpally and Vrinda Marwah explain, taking the example of India, that ART development may be seen as a threat for women's health, bodies and autonomy as well for recipients and donors, and as accentuating inequalities when there is no "protective barrier" to safeguard women's rights. Other chapters highlight the medical risk with, for instance, the transfer of multiple embryos leading to multiple births with the aim of increasing the chances of having a child (Zegers-Hochschild, Shah et al., Whittaker, Corrêa). However, the practice of multiple embryo transfer is commonly considered by the scientific community as more risky than single pregnancy, both for the parturient and the future baby. In Brazil, for instance, up to four embryos can be transferred.

Andrea Whittaker and Françoise Shenfield focus on the legal risks of transnational surrogacy, such as producing stateless and parentless children. Legal considerations can lead to difficulty in obtaining an entry or exit visa. They can result in either the absence of legal recognition of children or parents in their home country, or the absence of nationality attribution for the child. Andrea Whittaker points out legal risks in transnational surrogacy used by Australian nationals. Through four cases brought before the Family Court of Australia, she shows the complexity and dilemmas of banning or limiting its use. Françoise Shenfield examines the legal risks for British people seeking surrogacy abroad, and discusses some options for avoiding these risks (legislation or fair compensation, as for egg donation in some countries).

These concerns led some international medical associations (Shenfield et al., 2011; American Society for Reproductive Medicine, 2013a; 2013b) to promote new guidelines to safeguard the interests and ensure respect of all parties involved in the ART process. They advise an altruistic approach to surrogacy, managed by non-profit organisations, with special consideration for cross-border cases. The main recommendation made by Duru Shah, Sabahat Rasool and Nagadeepti Nagarajan at the end of their chapter on surrogacy in India is that a law should be voted and that it should be enforced.

ART as a gender issue

ART calls particular attention to gender issues, with a specific impact on women (Birenbaum-Carmeli, 2009). As the book shows, all over the world women are the main protagonists of ART treatments (Nadimpally and Marwah, Benabed, Birenbaum-Carmeli, Zegers-Hochschild, Corrêa). The male partner is often disregarded or absent during the medical process (de La Rochebrochard, 2003). In India, Sucharita Pujari and Sayeed Unisa found that women along with female relatives visit the clinics for treatment and the men usually lack basic knowledge about the reproductive organs, fertile period and diagnosis. Sarojini Nadimpally and Vrinda Marwah expressively speak about "no-man" in ART, as men do not even go to the first consultation and tests. Aicha Benabed shows throughout her chapter how much recourse to ART is painful and stressful for women in Algeria.

ART particularly deals with gender (in)equalities, exactly like every reproductive issue (Satz, 1992; Löwy, Rozée and Tain, 2014). It may in fact reaffirm the usual correlation between womanhood and motherhood and, therefore, reinforce patriarchal norms (Ragone and Twine, 2000; Thompson, 2002; Gupta, 2006). Marilena Corrêa considers that ART leads to a "naturalisation of motherhood", where the "desire to have a child and to set up a family [has become] a necessary logical piece". ART makes a mother, but it also makes "non-mothers", i.e. "non-women", which is deeply stigmatising all over the world, as we previously mentioned. But at the same time, ART may be seen as a reproductive empowerment, helping individuals and couples to have a child and, especially for women, to escape the usual stigmatisation attached to infertility and childlessness. However, we have to realise that the journey through ART may turn into a headlong rush forward. It may create a scenario where people will use ART for a child at any cost (Véronique Duchesne compared CBRC to biomedical roaming for women), often seen as lending itself to exploitation.

Gender issues are mostly highlighted in the current controversies and arguments regarding ART and the practice of surrogacy on the transnational scene. Some published studies discuss the exploitation attached to ART on the local and transnational scene (Corea, 1988; Donchin, 2010; Pfeffer, 2011). Andrea Whittaker presents five incidents of transnational surrogacy in Thailand, some of them dealing with female trafficking or exploitation. The present book focuses on the ambivalent impact of such practices on gender conditions. Surrogacy may be seen as both exploitation and empowerment, an escape route from poverty and stigmatisation (Rozée and Unisa, 2014). The ambivalence of surrogacy is well illustrated in the public debate in France, used as a starting point by Delphine Lance and Jennifer Merchant to discuss the ethnocentric nature of ethical critiques. Elly Teman, writing on surrogacy in Israel, shows that the practice is a positive experience for both surrogates and intended mothers; but she also states in her conclusion that what she observes in her country contrasts with what happens in India.

There is indeed a consensus that surrogates are at risk of exploitation due to differences in social and economic status between the women and the intended parents. Vulnerability is highest when surrogates come from less advantaged countries. Analysing weblogs and documentaries on transnational surrogacy in India, Karen Hvidtfeldt demonstrates that "Indian surrogates and Western prospective parents operate on unequal terms" regarding opportunities and status. Although there is evident risk in being a surrogate, Sharmila Rudrappa shows that for Indian women it may be an opportunity of empowerment. She observed that in Bangalore, surrogacy was described by the women themselves as a better option than their previous occupation. Surrogates are aware of the exploitative nature of their commitment. However, they opt for it for two reasons. Firstly, they face hard working conditions in the garment industry. Secondly, surrogacy offers more benefits, namely financial gains, better respect and decision-making in the family and satisfaction through helping a couple.

Social representation of ART

As we have said, cultural and religious representations of infertility and ART also reveal disparities and pluralism (Inhorn, 2003). The book shows that ART is an echo to social, cultural and religious norms (Benabed, Birenbaum-Carmeli, Zegers-Hochschild, Lance and Merchant), either encouraging or limiting use of the techniques.

As Daphna Birenbaum-Carmeli shows, in Israel infertile and childless women are seen as useless, disabled and selfish; reproduction, even through ART, is therefore encouraged (subject to certain religious conditions), but some techniques such as egg donation remain limited (also for religious reasons). In many countries, genetic kinship is socially valued and better accepted than social kinship through adoption. ART is in line with this preference, enabling genetic offspring. This may promote ART facilities in certain countries and explains why many parents seek such treatments rather than other alternatives.

ART also redefines, deconstructs and reconstructs family and parenting norms, which are generally and traditionally based on heterosexual union and intra-partnership reproduction (Chavkin and Maher, 2010; Tain, 2013; Rozée, 2015). Aicha Benabed explains that use of a third party for reproductive assistance is prohibited in Algeria, because this is not consistent with Islamic law. In Latin America, which is predominantly Catholic, procreation without reproductive sexual intercourse is not tolerated by Catholic tradition. Therefore, the weight of the Catholic church explains why there is no law on ART in the sub-continent (except in Argentina and Uruguay) and why it was even previously prohibited in some countries (see Zegers-Hochschild in this book). The social and cultural context explains why ART may be available, accepted or limited in many countries.

Many authors in this book underline the importance of the social context in understanding and analysing ART issues. They have observed that even when religion prohibits some practices, access or techniques, ways and means are often found to access ART and have a child. At the same time, even if a practice is legal, this does not mean that it is socially accepted. Indian surrogates, for instance, may face social and family disapproval, as shown in the chapter by Duru Shah, Sabahat Rasool and Nagadeepti Nagarajan. Delphine Lance and Jennifer Merchant show that Ukrainian and North American surrogates adapt and interact with the legal and social framework. Ukrainian surrogates, for instance, need approval from the church to engage in surrogacy. Surrogacy may be experienced negatively because of social disregard.

An interesting way to approach the social representation of ART is by exploring media and social networks (Thorn and Dill, 2010; Speier, 2011; Deonandan et al., 2012). In this book, Daphna Birenbaum-Carmeli, Karen Hvidtfeldt and Andrea Whittaker present analyses based on social media. These give an idea on how ART is perceived and (un)accepted in society and in restricted circles of society (or surrogacy users, in the case of Hvidtfeldt). Daphna Birenbaum-Carmeli looks at the way egg freezing in Israel has lately been presented in the media, analysing ten online articles in the daily press from 2008 to 2012. Karen Hvidtfeldt explores how surrogacy in India is described by Western intended parents and how it is shown in documentaries made by Western filmmakers. She demonstrates how the discourses of Western intended parents reflect globalisation and liberalistic logic, using "modern management rhetoric" (surrogates are for instance compared to "active entrepreneurs"). In documentaries, infertile individuals and couples are described as "legitimate consumers in the transnational reproductive economy".

Generally, the press has a worldwide stranglehold on ART issues, even transnational ones. This is demonstrated by the number of articles published on surrogacy in India in the international press over the last decade. As ART is very poorly studied in the developed world, the media are still the main source of information, dealing with sensational incidents. So drawing on field studies and scientific analysis, some chapters show the contrast between what we are commonly given to read or see and what really happens in some countries. An example is surrogacy in Bangalore (India), approached by Sharmila Rudrappa (see above). Elly Teman, in her study on surrogates in Israel, describes how surrogates feel distanced genetically and emotionally from the pregnancy (no maternal bond observed), and then proud of what they accomplish: they gave a baby to a woman who could not have one and they "made this other woman into a mother".

The press monopoly also highlights major events relating to ART practices, leading to new guidelines or laws. Transnational surrogacy between Australia and Thailand hit the headlines in recent years with the case of Baby Gammy (discussed in Whittaker's chapter). This led to international awareness of what really happens in Thailand and then to a new national law restricting access to surrogacy for foreigners.

Conclusion

From a multidisciplinary perspective and drawing on multisite studies, this book highlights some new issues relating to ART and discusses some older issues regarding infertility. ART is an increasing phenomenon irrespective of legal and political regulation. This is mainly because some people want a child "at any cost", even if procedures are not regulated or authorised in their home country. Nevertheless, available or legal does not mean accepted by society, and the converse is also true. But what this book clearly shows is that if there is no legislation, the medical and social risks are increased and inequalities between both national and international users are deepened.

Except for some points related to economic and political structures and opportunities, the commonalities and specificities of ART issues overstep the usual binary division of the world into South vs North or welfare states vs less developed countries. Each society faces these challenges against the background of their own historical, political, economic, cultural and religious background and norms. Globalisation, which makes exchanges and cross-border travel easier, the increasing medicalisation of reproduction and the related development of ART all raise new questions and confront societies with new challenges. These challenges may be local and specific, but the state-of-the-art analysis presented in this book shows that they are also global and common to all. This book opens, therefore, a new approach and a new scientific dialogue to deal with (un)common issues; it is our hope that it will lead to the further research that is greatly needed for a better understanding.

References

American Society for Reproductive Medicine. 2013a. Access to fertility treatment by gays, lesbians, and unmarried persons: a committee opinion, *Fertility and Sterility*, 100(6):1524–1527.

American Society for Reproductive Medicine. 2013b. Cross-border reproductive care: a committee opinion, *Fertility and Sterility*, 100(3):645–650.

Birenbaum-Carmeli, D. 2009. Contested surrogacy and the gender order: an Israeli case study, in Birenbaum-Carmeli, D. and Inhorn, M.C. (eds), *Assisting reproduction, testing genes. Global encounters with new biotechnologies*, New York: Berghahn Books, pp.189–210.

Chavkin, W., Maher, J.M. (eds). 2010. *The globalization of motherhood: deconstructions and reconstructions of biology and care*, New York: Routledge.

Cobo, A., Garcia-Velasco, J.A., Domingo, J., Remohí, J., Pellicer, A. 2013. Is vitrification of oocytes useful for fertility preservation for age-related fertility decline and in cancer patients?, *Fertility and Sterility*, 99(6):1485–1495.

Cobo, A., Garrido, N., Coello, A., Castello, D., Pellicer, A., Remohí, J. 2014. Cumulative live birth rates (CLBR) according to the number of vitrified oocytes consumed in an ovum donation (OD) egg-banking program, Communication, 30th ESHRE Annual Meeting, Munich, Germany, June 29–July 4.

Collins, J., Cook, J. 2010. Cross-border reproductive care: now and into the future, *Fertility and Sterility*, 94(1):25–26.

Corea, G. 1988 [1985]. *The mother machine: reproductive technologies from artificial insemination to artificial wombs*, New York: Harper and Row.

Crozier, G.K., Martin, D. 2012. How to address the ethics of reproductive travel to developing countries: a comparison of national self-sufficiency and regulated market approaches, *Developing World Bioethics*, 12:45–54.

de La Rochebrochard, E. 2003. Des hommes médicalement assistés pour procréer: IAD, FIV, ICSI, bilan d'une révolution dans la prise en charge médicale de l'infertilité masculine, *Population*, 58(4–5):549–586.

Deonandan, R., Loncar, M., Rahman, P., Omar, S. 2012. Measuring reproductive tourism through an analysis of Indian ART clinic websites, *International Journal of General Medicine*, 5:763–773.

Donchin, A. 2010. Reproductive tourism and the quest for global gender justice, *Bioethics*, 24:323–332.

Dondorp, W., de Wert, G., Pennings, G., Shenfield, F., Devroey, P., Tarlatzis, B., Barri, P., Diedrich, K. 2012. ESHRE Task Force on Ethics and Law, 2012, Oocyte cryopreservation for age-related fertility loss, *Human Reproduction*, 27(5):1231–1237.

Ferraretti, A.P., Pennings, G., Gianaroli, L., Natali, F., Magli, M.C. 2010. Cross-border reproductive care: a phenomenon expressing the controversial aspects of reproductive technologies, *Reproductive Biomedicine Online*, 20:261–266.

Gupta, J.A. 2006. Toward transnational feminism: some reflections and concerns in relation to the globalization of reproductive technologies, *European Journal of Women's Studies*, 13:23–38.

Gürtin, Z.B., Inhorn, M.C. 2011. Introduction: travelling for conception and the global assisted reproduction market, *Reproductive Biomedicine Online*, 23:535–537.

Hudson, N., Culley, L., Blyth, E., Norton, W., Rapport, F., Pacey, A. 2011. Cross-border reproductive care: a review of the literature, *Reproductive Biomedicine Online*, 22:673–685.

Inhorn, M.C. 2003. *Local babies, global science: gender, religion, and in vitro fertilization in Egypt*, New York: Routledge.

Inhorn, M.C. 2004. Middle Eastern masculinities in the age of new reproductive technologies: Male infertility and stigma in Egypt and Lebanon, *Medical Anthropology Quarterly*, 18(2):162–182.

Inhorn, M.C. 2009. Right to assisted reproductive technology: overcoming infertility in low-resource countries, *International Journal of Gynecology and Obstetrics*, 106:172–174.

Inhorn, M.C., Gürtin, Z.B. 2011. Cross-border reproductive care: a future research agenda, *Reproductive Biomedicine Online*, 23:665–676.

Inhorn, M.C., van Balen, F. (eds). 2002. *Infertility around the globe: new thinking on childlessness, gender and reproductive technologies*, Berkeley: University of California Press.

Jejeebhoy, S.J. 1998. Infertility in India – levels, patterns and consequences: priorities for social science research, *Journal of Family Welfare*, 44(2):15–24.

Löwy, I., Rozée, V., Tain, L. 2014. Nouvelles techniques reproductives, nouvelle production du genre (Introduction) [New reproductive techniques, new gender production (Introduction)], *Cahiers du Genre*, 56:5–18.

Nachtigall, R.D. 2006. International disparities in access to infertility services, *Fertility and Sterility*, 85(4):871–875.

Nahman, M.R. 2013. *Extractions. An Ethnography of Reproductive Tourism*, Basingstoke: Palgrave Macmillan, Global Ethics Series.

Pennings, G. 2004. Legal harmonization and reproductive tourism in Europe, *Human Reproduction*, 19:2689–2694.

Pfeffer, N. 2011. Eggs-ploiting women: a critical feminist analysis of the different principles in transplant and fertility tourism, *Reproductive Biomedicine Online*, 23:634–641.

Ragone, H., Twine F.W. (eds). 2000. *Ideologies and technologies of motherhood: race, class, sexuality, nationalism*, New York: Routledge.

Rozée, V. 2011. L'AMP sans frontière [ART without borders], *Bulletin Epidémiologique Hebdomadaire*, 23–24:270–273.

Rozée, V. 2015. Les normes de la maternité en France à l'épreuve du recours transnational de l'assistance médicale à la procréation, *Recherches Familiales*, 12:43–55.

Rozée, V., de La Rochebrochard, E. 2013. Cross-border reproductive care among French patients: experiences in Greece, Spain and Belgium, *Human Reproduction*, 28(11):3103–3110.

Rozée, V., Mazuy M. 2012. L'infertilité dans les couples hétérosexuels: genre et "gestion" de l'échec, *Sciences Sociales et Santé*, 30(4):5–29.

Rozée, V., Unisa S. 2014. Surrogacy from reproductive rights perspective: the case of India, *Autrepart*, 70(2):185–203.

Rudrappa, S. 2010. Making India the 'mother destination': outsourcing labor to Indian surrogates, in Williams, C. and Dellinger, K. (eds), *Gender and Sexuality in the Workplace, Research in the Sociology of Work*, 20:253–285.

SAMA Team. 2007. Assisted reproductive technologies in India: implications for women, *Economic & Political Weekly*, 42(23):2184–2189.

Satz, D. 1992. Markets in women's reproductive labor, *Philosophy and Public Affairs*, 21(2):107–131.

Sen, A. 1990. Gender and cooperative conflicts, in Tinker, I. (ed.), *Persistent inequalities: women and world development*, New York: Oxford University Press, 458–500.

Shenfield F., de Mouzon, J., Pennings, G., Ferraretti, A.P., Nyboe Anderson, A., de Wert, G., Goossens, V., on behalf of the ESHRE Task Force 'Cross-Border Reproductive Care' (CBRC). 2010. Cross-border reproductive care in six European countries, *Human Reproduction*, 25(6):1361–1368.

Shenfield, F., Pennings, G., de Mouzon, J., Ferraretti, A.P., Goossens, V., on behalf of the ESHRE Task Force 'Cross-Border Reproductive Care' (CBRC). 2011. ESHRE's good practice guide for cross-border reproductive care for centers and practitioners, *Human Reproduction*, 26:1625–1627.

Speier, A.R. 2011. Brokers, consumers and the internet: how North American consumers navigate their infertility journeys, *Reproductive Biomedicine Online*, 23:592–599.

Storrow, R.F. 2006. Quests for conception: fertility tourists, globalization, and feminist legal theory, *Hastings Law Journal*, 57:295–330.

Storrow, R.F. 2010. The pluralism problem in cross-border reproductive care, *Human Reproduction*, 25(12):2939–2943.

Tain, L. 2013. *Le corps reproducteur. Dynamiques de genre et pratiques reproductives*, Rennes: Presses de l'EHESP.

Thompson C. 2002. Fertile ground: feminists theorize infertility, in Inhorn, M.C. and van Balen, F. (eds), *Infertility around the globe: new thinking on childlessness, gender and reproductive technologies*, Berkeley: University of California Press, 52–78.

Thorn, P., Dill, S. 2010. The role of patients' organizations in cross-border reproductive care, *Fertility and Sterility*, 94:23–24.

Unisa, S. 1999. Childlessness in Andhra Pradesh, India: treatment-seeking and consequences, *Reproductive Health Matters*, 7(13):54–64.

Whittaker, A. 2011. Cross-border assisted reproduction care in Asia: implications for access, equity and regulations, *Reproductive Health Matters*, 19:107–116.

Zegers-Hochschild, F., Adamson, G.D., de Mouzon, J., Ishihara, O., Mansour, R., Nygren, K., Sullivan, E., Vanderpoel, S., for ICMART and WHO. 2009. International Committee for Monitoring Assisted Reproductive Technology (ICMART) and the World Health Organization (WHO) revised glossary of ART terminology, 2009, *Fertility and Sterility*, 92(5):1520–1524.

Part I

ART regulation and journey

1 Access to ARTs in Latin America

Fernando Zegers-Hochschild

Introduction

Infertility is "a disease of the reproductive system defined by the failure to achieve a clinical pregnancy after 12 months or more of regular unprotected sexual intercourse" (Zegers-Hochschild et al., 2009; 2010).

The World Health Organization (WHO) together with the International Committee Monitoring Assisted Reproductive Technology (ICMART) defined infertility as a disease, acknowledging that it can severely impact the health of individuals as well as their families; unfortunately, the majority of countries in the developing world still consider infertility a matter of personal desires and therefore, when allocating human and economic resources to health priorities, infertility does not compete with other diseases affecting women's health. Priorities are therefore placed on adolescent pregnancies and global strategies directed towards fertility regulation programs, leaving the problem of infertility as the last priority.

Infertility is a disease that has diverse effects on physical and psychological health, as well as social consequences, including marital instability, anxiety, depression, social isolation and loss of social status, loss of gender identity, ostracism and abuse. Most religions attribute great value to families with numerous children. Thus, infertility also affects religious well-being in life and for some communities, even after death (Dyer, 2007; Van Balen and Bos, 2009). To a certain extent, these consequences find their origin in the fact that, particularly in developing countries, infertility violates the social norm that having many children is a blessing. The transgression of this norm, although unintended, creates stigmatization. Socially, infertile woman and men carry less value as persons, and in turn, infertile women and men feel less valuable than those who have children. This leads to a systematic loss of self-esteem, which has consequences in multiple spheres of the personal and social life of those with this illness. Social, psychological and cultural consequences of infertility have been classified into six levels of severity, ranging from feelings of guilt, fear and depression to loss of dignity and death due to violence and suicide (Daar and Merali, 2002).

Magnitude of the problem

Population studies estimate that at least 10% of women in reproductive years suffer from infertility. This is equivalent to approximately 80 million couples in the world (Boivin et al., 2007), and almost 14,000,000 in Latin America. The prevalence of primary infertility has increased in developed countries as well as in emerging economies due to postponement of childbearing resulting from the dilemma that many women face: trying to harmonize their reproductive wishes with their personal growth in other aspects of their academic, work and social life.

Paradoxically, many developing countries have both overpopulation problems and infertility. Infertile couples in these countries are severely affected since they are socially marginalized by their families and communities, as well as by health systems that do not recognize the need to provide support in terms of economic and technical resources for people suffering from this type of disease.

Inequality in the access to fertility treatments

Rich and poor nations around the world have committed themselves to providing reproductive healthcare to their people. As early as 1994, at the Conference on Population and Development held in Cairo, 180 nations recognized and agreed that reproductive health was part of the concept of global health, and governments agreed on a program of action that included providing universal access to reproductive health services. Prevention and treatment of infertility were explicitly recognized as part of the challenges concerning reproductive health. Less than ten years later, in 2001, nations made an even more demanding commitment, and set forth the Millennium Development Goals (MDG). The absence of infertility treatments is a relevant barrier to universal access to reproductive health (MDG5), and constitutes a source of inequality concerning the access to benefits available through science and technology.

Rich and poor people are equally deserving of reproduction, and people suffering from infertility deserve access to health as much as people suffering from other diseases. The lack of access to effective and safe treatments is a source of discrimination between rich and poor people in all developing countries. Many countries find excuses for this social injustice, arguing a high rate of population growth. However, barriers to fertility treatments due to economic, political, ethno-social and religious reasons mainly affect infertile and poor people, since people with economic and social resources can always afford to cover treatment (out of pocket-funding and/or travel to other countries) and receive more modern, safer and more effective treatments.

Throughout the world, the availability of infertility services is the result of public health policies associated with a variety of socio-economic, political and, in many cases, religious influences. Wide disparities exist in the access, quality and delivery of infertility services within developed countries, but most of all between developed and developing countries. Relatively few members of the world's infertile population have complete equitable access to the full range of infertility treatment at affordable levels. Even in wealthy countries, such as the United States, access to assisted reproductive technology (ART) is, or has been, marked by high disparity and inequality in the access to treatment, partly due to high costs and legislative decisions.

In countries where access to infertility treatment is granted by law, fertility is understood as a right to which all women and men are entitled in equal conditions. The provision of egalitarian access to fertility treatments such as ART is also followed by regulations restricting women's autonomy, such as decisions on age limits or the number of embryos to be transferred, among others. The purpose of these limitations is to include as many couples requiring treatment as possible.

On the other hand, when access to infertility treatment is not part of a governmental policy, individuals must rely on their personal wealth and/or private insurance covering medical care. The vast majority of institutions providing ART treatment in the Americas do so in the absence of a national or private funding system. A study commissioned by RESOLVE, the National Infertility Association of the United States, to Mercer Health and Benefits in 2006 (www.resolve.org) showed that approximately 80% of treatments provided in the United States are pocket-funded, and the same applies to Latin America (see www.redlara.com), where the vast majority of institutions providing treatment are private centers. Under this scenario, the regulation of access to diagnosis and treatment is left to a free market policy, leaving out of reach all those who cannot afford the costs involved. Furthermore, in most countries in Latin America, companies providing private health insurance do not cover the costs involved in the treatment of infertility.

Coverage of infertility treatments offers some additional difficulties. While nobody would question the use of all available tools in order to save the lives of people with cancer, the use of modern reproductive technology is controversial and many legislators wonder whether specific treatments should be available or funded in order to generate a new life. Interestingly, there is much more social acceptance and legislative agreement in saving lives than in generating new ones.

Of course, those promoting laws and regulations have already been born; all they need to worry about is the quality of their aging and death. On the other hand, for those who have not yet come into existence, there is no chance to influence policymakers unless the latter have experienced infertility or been emotionally moved by someone with this condition.

The purpose of this chapter is to examine ART in Latin America from the perspective of access to treatment and how this impacts the way treatment is performed.

ART in Latin America

ART has been practiced in Latin America since the early eighties, and the first baby born from ART was born in 1984. Since 1990, most institutions providing treatment in the region have joined the Latin American Registry of ART (RedLara: www.redlara.com). This registry gathers individualized data from 160 institutions in 12 countries in the region. The information available includes individualized data from the start of a cycle until birth or miscarriage. This registry has made it possible to look at regional trends over the years as well as biomedical, epidemiologic and cultural markers of access to treatment as well as the safety and efficacy of different treatment alternatives (Zegers-Hochschild et al., 2014).

The vast majority of countries in Latin America have not officially recognized infertility as a disease; therefore, this condition remains ignored as a public health need. Also, due to the intervention of conservative groups, ART, although not prohibited, is not officially registered as an accepted treatment. Therefore, infertile couples cannot count on public or private health insurance to cover infertility treatments. These conservative groups, very much in accordance with the Catholic Magisterium, argue that ART constitutes a threat to human life, embodied in the embryo. Therefore, most ART procedures are carried out in private institutions, generating inequality in access and leaving many infertile couples devoid of medical treatment. So far, Argentina and Uruguay are the only countries in Latin America with laws regulating access to ART. Both laws make specific reference to the ICMART/WHO definition of infertility as a disease, and establish that access should be granted to women or couples with no discrimination in terms of their sexual preferences or economic capacity. Furthermore, after the ruling of the Inter-American Court of Human Rights, Costa Rica has been forced to pass a law making ART available to all citizens (Zegers-Hochschild et al., 2013) over the years. Although the Court does not refer to specific conditions such as single women or same-sex couples, the intention is to avoid discrimination on the grounds of financial incapacity. The law is not yet approved in Costa Rica, and there are strong disagreements centered on whether embryo freezing and gamete donation should be included in the law.

One of the consequences of the absence of national regulatory bodies is that important decisions are left uncontrolled: the number of embryos to be transferred, the age limit for undergoing oocyte donation (OD), anonymity of donors, economic compensation and access to treatment for same-sex couples and single women, etc. There are regional guidelines provided by RedLara as well as national guidelines provided by scientific societies, but none of these are enforceable except in Argentina and Uruguay, which now have laws regulating access to ART and, to a certain extent, how ART should be performed.

When access is expressed as the number of ART cycles per million women of reproductive age (for the purpose of this calculation we have considered women between 25 and 40 years), the proportion of treatment cycles fluctuates between 17,000 and 23,000 cycles per million women of reproductive age in Scandinavian countries such as Sweden and Denmark, and between 5,000 and 7,000 cycles in the UK and Germany. The disproportion is even greater between European countries and other regions of the world. Using the same calculations, access in the United States is 3,000 cycles per million, while access to ART treatments in countries in Latin American such as Argentina, Brazil and Chile drops to between 400 and 1,000 cycles per million.

There is a close relationship between socio-economic policies concerning access to infertility treatments on the one hand, and the way patients and their health providers ponder risks and benefits on the other. In countries where treatment is provided by national funds, as in the Scandinavian countries, Israel and Australia, among others, the mean number of embryos transferred is under two. Instead, in countries where the cost of treatment is regulated by the market and access is restricted to those who can afford high costs, the number of embryos transferred is much higher, thus contributing to multiple births. The proportion of multiple births and high-order multiple births in Brazil is 22.6% and 4.2% respectively, while in Sweden it drops to 4.6% and 0.1% respectively. This effect of market-regulated access to health is not limited to developing countries. In the United States, the proportion of twin pregnancies is even higher than in Latin America (29.8%), and constitutes 1.7% of high-order multiples in spite of the fact that many states authorize embryo reduction (Ishihara et al., 2007).

The influence of tradition and the Catholic Church

It is often difficult to measure the extent of the influence of religion, tradition and other cultural factors on the way laws regulate reproductive health. Except for some Islamic communities where religious leaders directly decide what is and what is not to be done, in many occidental societies religious morality permeates society and legislation through the promotion of their direct magisterium. However, the Catholic Church exerts much of its influence indirectly through economic and political alliances.

Although Christian religions and public laws have been separated for centuries in countries in Western Europe and the Americas, Christianity, and most of all the Roman Catholic Church, is by far the most outspoken religious body when it comes to moral behavior concerning sex and reproduction. Catholic tradition has a strong influence in Latin America, less in the United States, and even though most European countries have a more rational approach to morality in reproductive health issues, the Catholic tradition can still exert strong influence. A recent example was the Italian law regulating the practice of ART. In May 2009 the Italian Constitutional Court declared that some parts of Article 14 of Law 40/2004 were "unconstitutional". In this way, the new law prohibited the insemination of more than three embryos. Embryo cryopreservation and OD were prohibited. This law was later modified for a more permissive approach to reproductive decisions.

The fundamental basis for the Catholic opposition to any form of ART began in the late 1960s, when Pope Paul VI established in his encyclical *Humane Vitae* that the uniting and procreative meanings of the conjugal act (coitus) should not be voluntarily dissociated. Consequently, both sex deliberately devoid of procreation and procreation without sex are even today considered immoral as they voluntarily dissociate these two meanings one by allowing sexual intercourse devoid of its procreative meaning, the other by allowing procreation not mediated by sexual intercourse. Later, in 1987, the Vatican published a document, *Donum Vitae*, which contained an "Instruction on respect for human life", issued by the Congregation for the doctrine of faith and signed by Cardinal Joseph Ratzinger, who later became Pope Benedictus XVI. This document stated that a life, as we understand it, exists from conception onwards, and therefore condemned all forms of assisted reproduction, irrespective of its intention, the source of gametes and marital status.[1] This principle carried such power that later, the vast majority of countries in the Americas signed the American Convention on Human Rights, Pact of Costa Rica,[2] which states in Article 4.1 that "laws should protect the lives of those to be born – in general from conception onwards". This concept of protection of those to be born is not included in the equivalent Article 2 of the European Convention of Human Rights, which refers exclusively to the right to life of actual persons. The inclusion of this right to protection of embryos/fetuses has opened enormous discussions, which have to do with the extent of this protection. For the more fundamental and conservative groups, this protection is equivalent to the right to life as an actual living person. For others, only actual living people have a right to life, and before birth the rights belong to the pregnant woman and the embryo's right to protection is always expressed through her rights. Adding the protection of embryos from conception often constitutes the substance of reproductive rights debates. One example is the penalization of the interruption of pregnancy. Four countries in Latin America (Chile, Nicaragua, El Salvador and Dominican Republic) still have laws penalizing every form of interruption of pregnancy, while the rest of Latin America, with the exception of Cuba, have very restrictive laws. The reason used is that the embryo/fetus is entitled to the right to life and should never be considered less deserving of the right to life when confronted with the rights of its mother.

Based on Article 4.1 of the Inter-American Convention of Human Rights, the Supreme Court of Costa Rica stopped ART under the basis of the constitutional obligation to protect human embryos. In the rest of Latin America, ART is performed, but no laws were available until Argentina and Uruguay managed to overcome the influence of Catholicism. Many other countries, however, have law projects sitting in their parliaments. In the majority of cases, this is mainly because no agreements have been reached between legislators as to whether pre-implantation embryos are entitled to rights of their own. Needless to say, different forms of embryo manipulation, genetic diagnosis or research are performed in several Latin American countries without the possibility of discarding abnormal embryos.

The influence of Catholicism concerning ART is less evident in the United States, where more value is placed on the right to autonomy, from the perspective of both couples and providers. It must be said, however, that the opposition of the US government to therapeutic cloning and embryonic stem cell research, which lasted until President Obama was elected, was mainly the result of lobbying by the Catholic Church under the argument that a pre-implantation embryo is entitled to the same rights as an existing person.

For various reasons, the Council of Bishops in Europe has been more liberal in the application of directives arising from the Vatican. An example is the Catholic University of Leuven, Belgium, where ART, including embryo cryopreservation, is offered openly. A reverse example, however, is the recent law passed in Italy which forbids fertilization of more than three oocytes, embryo cryopreservation, use of donor gametes, genetic diagnosis, etc. The reason behind this restrictive law is the result of pressure from the Catholic Church on the basis of human rights attributable to embryos from conception onwards.[3]

In a different attitude towards reproduction, Protestant denominations (Baptist, Methodist, Lutheran, Mormon, Presbyterian, Episcopalian and others) are very liberal concerning infertility treatments and the promotion of reproductive science. ART is accepted as long as gametes belong to spouses and there is no intention of destroying embryos.

The purpose of reviewing religious morality is that, especially in the developing world, religion can have a strong influence on political decisions. In countries dominated by Catholic tradition, which today are concentrated mainly in Latin America, much of the discussion is not centered on the rights of infertile women and men. On the contrary, most of the discussion is centered on the moral rights of an embryo. As a consequence of the above, ART is accepted because it is there, but only two countries (Argentina and Uruguay) have been able to reach a consensus on minimal standards to regulate the practice of ART in order to make it universally available. This lack of pragmatism in confronting biomedical and social realities is at least in part responsible for the low access to treatment generating inequality, lack of autonomy and therefore absence of diagnostic and therapeutic procedures, such as pre-implantation genetic diagnosis (PGD) and other forms of preventing the inheritance of genetic diseases. In countries where the influence of religion in public policies has been restricted, it is the right of persons that prevails in as much as it does not affect society as a whole.

It is my understanding that the more separation there is as to how and who is entitled to impose religious and public laws, the more respect there is for the needs of women, men and unborn children.

Societies strongly influenced by religious moralities tend to defend their moral principles over the always-changing needs of their people. On the other hand, societies built upon pragmatic and secularly based political structures tend to base their regulatory bodies on what people recognize as their needs, respecting the autonomy that rules individual lives.

Final remarks

Infertility generates a number of complex feelings such as anguish, depression and isolation and weakens family ties, particularly in societies that value the size of the family above all. Women who cannot "give her husband a son" are regarded as odd beings who "must have done something wrong to be unworthy of such a blessing". On the other hand, men who cannot father a son are also regarded as less "macho". An interesting study from Harvard University shows that when emotional characteristics of women diagnosed with infertility are compared with a control group equivalent in socio-demographic variables, there is a greater prevalence and predictability of depression in the infertile group. Infertile women present a higher incidence of depressive symptomatology, and their levels of anxiety and depression are only comparable to women with pathologies such as coronary disease, cancer or HIV (Domar, 1992).

Based on the abundant scientific evidence showing the psychosocial deterioration caused by infertility, it is hard to believe that people living with this disease will feel indifferent about having access to treatment or having treatment denied for economic and/or moral reasons.

Poor women suffering from infertility are heavily punished, in the first place because they cannot have access to treatment, unlike other women who will be treated if the cause of their infertility is amenable to treatment by acceptable and cheaper interventions such as hormone stimulation and intra-uterine insemination; second, because in most of Latin America, only a minority of couples can afford treatment or travel abroad, generating social inequality; and third, because in addition to being denied treatment, those who undergo treatments are stigmatized by some of the most conservative religious communities. This was the case in Costa Rica, where the Constitutional Court determined in the year 2000 that IVF was an attempt against the right to life of human beings (embryos). Newspapers, television and radio programs referred to those receiving IVF treatments as being responsible for the death of many. Today, right-wing Catholic organizations, such as Opus Dei, express public opposition and condemn any form of ART.

More and more, women and men in Latin America are advocating for their autonomy when deciding on reproductive and sexual rights. This proved to be possible in Argentina and Uruguay, and several countries in the Caribbean are about to follow.

Indeed, the recognition of the right to start a family as a human right has meant a large step forward, but there is still a long way to go in order to prioritize ART in the health agenda in countries in Latin America.

Notes

1 Congregación para la Doctrina y la Fe, Vaticano. *Instrucción Donum Vitae Sobre el respeto a la vida humana naciente y la dignidad de la procreación, 1987.*
2 American Convention of Human Rights. Pact of San Jose de Costa Rica, 1969 (B-32).
3 Since the time of writing, this is no longer the case.

References

Boivin, J, Bunting, L, Collins, JA, Nygren, KG. 2007. *International estimates of infertility prevalence and treatment-seeking: potential need and demand for infertility medical care.* Hum Reprod 22(6):1506–1512.

Daar, M, Merali, Z. 2002. *Infertility and assisted reproductive technologies in the developing world.* In: Current Practices and Controversies in Assisted Reproduction, Vayena, E, Rowe, PJ, Griffin, PD (eds). Geneva: WHO.

Domar, A. 1992. *The prevalence and predictability of depression in infertile women.* Fertil and Steril 1158–1163.

Dyer, SJ. 2007. *The value of children in African countries – Insights from studies on infertility.* J Psychosom Obstets & Gynaecol 28(2):69–77.

Ishihara, O, Adamson, GD, Dyer, S, de Mouzon, J, Nygren, KG, Sullivan, EA, Zegers-Hochschild, F, Mansour, R. 2007. *International Committee for Monitoring Assisted Reproductive Technologies: World Report on Assisted Reproductive Technologies, 2007.* Fertil and Steril 103(2):402–413.

Van Balen, F, Bos, HMW. 2009. *The social and cultural consequences of being childless in poor resource areas.* FV&V in ObGYN 1(2):106–121.

Zegers-Hochschild, F, Adamson, GD, de Mouzon, J, Ishihara, O, Mansour, R, Nygren, K, Sullivan, E, Van Der Poel, S. 2009. International Committee for Monitoring Assisted Reproductive Technology; World Health Organization. *The International Committee for Monitoring Assisted Reproductive Technology (ICMART) and the World Health Organization (WHO) Revised Glossary on ART Terminology, 2009.* Hum Reprod 24(11):2683–2687.

Zegers-Hochschild, F, Adamson, GD, de Mouzon, J, Ishihara, O, Mansour, R, Nygren, K, Sullivan, E, Van Der Poel, S. 2010. *Glosario de terminología en Técnicas de Reproducción Asistida (TRA).* Versión revisada y preparada por el International Committee for Monitoring Assisted Reproductive Technology (ICMART) y la Organización Mundial de la Salud (OMS). Traducido y Publicado por la Red Latinoamericana de Reproducción Asistida en 2010.

Zegers-Hochschild, F, Dickens, BM, Dughman-Manzur, S. 2013. Human rights to in vitro fertilization. *International Journal of Gynecology and Obstetrics* 123(1):86–89.

Zegers-Hochschild, F, Schwarze, JE, Crosby, JA, Musri, C, do Carmo Borges de Souza, M. 2014. *Assisted Reproductive Technology in Latin America: the Latin American Registry, 2012.* RBM Online DOI: http://dx.doi.org/10.1016/j.rbmo.2014.10.003.

2 ARTs in Brazil

Public and private arrangements in the name of access and reproductive rights

Marilena C. D. V. Corrêa

Introduction

How can a woman live without children in contemporary societies where, in the last 35 to 40 years, techniques for producing babies on demand have emerged? This is an especially valid question in contexts such as the Brazilian one, where having a child is a highly valued social norm, and motherhood is still identified as a natural female condition. Regardless of this naturalization of motherhood, human reproduction concerns the reproduction of individuals situated in social positions, entailing the constitution of families, forming and regulating kinship relations, transmitting names, symbolic and cultural heritage, education and socialization. Hence, it goes far beyond the mere procreative aspect of biological conception.

Yet, although presented and represented as a technological revolution landmark in medicine today, ART can be seen as the latest stage in a process of continuous medical intervention on reproduction and women's bodies. The medicalization of childlessness through ART is not a break in a medical and social tradition that had already developed technological birth control (with powerful hormonal contraception). When ART emerged, the notion that having a child could (and even should) be an autonomous, controlled project, rationally managed through medical goods and services, was already established.

Indeed, the medicalization of childlessness is related to people's reproductive projects (Becker & Nachtigall, 1992), but it can also be approached from other perspectives: scientific interest; sale of medical services; production and liberation of human biological and reproductive material; population control; enhancement of the quality of human genetic pool; and North–South circulation of people in need of a child or reproductive material. That said, clinical reproductive medicine turned the desire to have a baby and set up a family into *a necessary piece of logic* when framing these techniques, regardless of infertility diagnosis (Corrêa, 1997).

The dissemination of ARTs in Brazil in the early 1980s, at first exclusively in private healthcare, was not accompanied by a legal and ethical framework to regulate these practices, thus making room for controversial interventions in women's bodies. Sensationalist media coverage, poor records and limited scientific evaluation of ART results also contributed to overshadowing their dubious effects on women's health. The first part of this chapter retells this history of ART in Brazil from the early 1980s to the late 1990s. From the 2000s on, ART monitoring initiatives in Latin America were undertaken, mainly by a regional professional society, the *Rede latino-americana de reprodução assistida*, and partially by official institutions such as Anvisa (the Brazilian regulatory health surveillance agency), as described in the second part of this chapter. To illustrate ongoing contradictions in ART commercialization today in Brazil, the last part of this chapter focuses on two current cases: the "Access Initiative", sponsored by international pharmaceutical companies in partnership with some local private clinics; and "shared oocyte donation". It analyzes the health, legal and normative issues, as well as the ethical and social dilemmas raised by such cases, in the context of moral conflict, vulnerability and unequal access to ART in the Global North and South.

The emergence of ART in Brazil

The birth of the first Brazilian test-tube baby was announced in 1984. From the early 1980s, IVF attempts were reported in Brazilian scientific journals, always recommending its effectiveness and the easy handling of the technique. Also in 1984, but before the IVF "success", a Brazilian medical group signed a contract with the biggest local broadcasting company, *Globo*, to finance the scientific mission of Australian doctors who traveled to train a small group of Brazilian doctors. The anticipated result, the first Brazilian test-tube baby, was to be broadcast, with copyrights being assigned to *Globo*. The project was abandoned because, before the anticipated IVF "triumph", a patient died due to complications following IVF procedures in the same clinic (Corea, 1985; Reis, 1987).

It is noteworthy that previous complex biomedical innovations (such as heart transplants and hemodialysis) were transferred either to universities or large public hospitals because of the very high costs of technological research and application; additionally, these were the institutions where most of the country's qualified staff was concentrated. Contrary to this innovation circuit, ART entered the country exclusively through private medicine, and even today almost 90% of the clinics offering such services are in private healthcare (Souza, 2014).

This is also true for professional training. From the 1980s, small private clinics financed courses and seminars to acquire know-how on techniques straight from foreign specialists. So-called "voluntary women", who normally could not afford their treatment, were enrolled in ART "research" programs in private clinics (mostly in the city of São Paulo), despite the concentration of specialized and postgraduate studies in public university centers. Generally, these women were hospitalized to undergo IVF under the supervision of foreign specialists, their resulting pregnancies being followed by Brazilian doctors. The two British specialists and the French doctor who participated in the first successful test-tube-baby projects in their respective countries came to Brazil, along with the Australian team which pioneered IVF worldwide. In my PhD research, the medical doctors interviewed in Rio de Janeiro and São Paulo evoked this scientific exchange "model" in the making of Brazilian reproductive medicine. Based on learning from foreign specialists and through hands-on methods applied to poor female volunteers, ART was soon available in private healthcare for upper strata patients willing to reproduce (Corrêa, 1997).

In private healthcare, test-tube babies became popular under rather specific circumstances: media coverage gave social visibility to IVF and its byproducts (frozen embryos, egg donations, pre-implantation diagnosis, sex selection, embryo triage). They were featured in the plot of soap operas,[1] a major television pastime in Brazil, and thus were broadcast in a sketchy way that did not unveil their controversial effects. ART was pictured as a remedy for natural handicaps, a simple response to the demand for babies reinforcing the social value of biological/genetic links. Failure in the application of different techniques and procedures, risks and even costs were rarely featured during the first 10 to 15 years of ART diffusion.

In the scientific and sanitary fields, it was also a time of little transparency due to low ART monitoring by both public and private health systems. The inadequate monitoring of ART results was addressed only in the mid-1990s, with the publication of the first Brazilian Report on ART (Franco & Wheba, 1994) by the Brazilian Society for Assisted Reproduction (*Sociedade Brasileira de Reprodução Assistida*), which gathered data and started a periodic record of ART results. However, data remained rare and underreported. For instance, while this report listed 14 IVF centers, the same specialists claimed 80 centers throughout the country in the media.

Still, the nonexistence of official institutions licensing clinics, the lack of records and the control of results created blind spots in ART monitoring in Brazil. The lack of political will among public health authorities paved the way for a non-regulated application of these techniques, which in turn lessened the critical capacity of Brazilian scientists to evaluate its use.

By the late 1990s, international literature already demonstrated that ARTs were not always efficient and imposed high costs and risks to women (Corrêa, 2000). These sanitary and scientific deficiencies challenge women's health and reproductive rights, and deepen their vulnerability to reproduction impairments.

Concerning the broader political context, where the early diffusion of ART and its impacts on access arose, 1988 was a landmark year in the political history of Brazil. After 24 years of military dictatorship, a Constituent Assembly of deputies elected by citizens issued a new democratic constitution. Following the Health Reform Movement (*Movimento Sanitarista*), set up by different civil and professional associations (health reform activists, feminists, labor unions), the constitution states that "Health is a right of the citizen and a duty of the State". Two years later, a law (Law 8080, passed on September 19, 1990) created the National Public Healthcare System (*Sistema Único de Saúde* – SUS), grounded on the principle of universal access to healthcare.[2]

With growing financing difficulties (budget cuts imposed by 1980s austerity policies), an increasing gap between SUS' costs and funding widened permanently. Nevertheless, SUS assured access to highly complex procedures, such as dialysis, cancer and HIV/AIDS treatment. This is not the case for ART, thus making it a controversial matter, since the Brazilian constitution opted for a broad definition of health (not only the absence of disease). Childlessness has not been prioritized and targeted by the public health budget. The unregulated context of ART application is both cause and effect of this controversy, as we will see below.

Towards regulation of ART

The first official resolution on ART was issued in 1992 by the Federal Council of Medicine (*CFM*, acronym in Portuguese) and dealt with licensing medical activities and regulating deontological matters through the issuing of normative resolutions. Resolution 1358 (and its 2010 and 2013 revisions) was the first and so far the only piece of regulation dealing specifically with ART. Nevertheless, other legal or non-statutory norms may affect ART since, for instance, the Brazilian Federal Constitution establishes that selling any parts of the human body is a criminal offense.

The CFM Resolution defined itself as an *ethical* document stemming from considerations on the legitimacy of the desire to overcome "human infertility – a health problem that holds medical and psychological implications" (op. cit., p. 1), while reaffirming the principles of non-commercialization of the human body or its parts, tissues and cells. According to the Federal Constitution, as well as the Law on Transplants (Law 9434, 1997), donation must not involve any form of payment or remuneration and must be anonymous. Moreover, donors must renounce any information about the use of their samples, including those regarding possible parenthood. Medical secrecy shall be respected, except in medical necessities, such as transplants, when information may be disclosed, if possible without civil identification of the donor.

Informed consent is mandatory. In fact, a single woman or a man, regardless of sexual orientation, may use ART, provided she or he agrees through informed consent. In the case of a couple, the consent of the partner is binding. Surrogacy ("temporary donation of the uterus") is also allowed, stressing that it should remain within the family circle, preferably within two "degrees". In any case, no remuneration shall exist.

Considering the near unavailability of IVF practice in public healthcare, the apparent arrangements for a universal eligibility are de facto related to the market and to consumers' purchasing power. The liberal approach of the CFM Resolution is not a real statement for fostering access.

The 2013 revision of the CFM Resolution explicitly mentions two important decisions of the Brazilian Supreme Court on homosexual couples and their recognition as a family unit. Although these Courts' decisions were not raised by ART concerns, only a few months later CFM changed its previous decision to explicitly legitimate what private clinics and doctors had been doing for years: using ART despite the sexual orientation of patients (who could afford it).

Regarding the maximum number of embryos to be transferred, the 2013 Resolution still admits the transfer of up to four embryos. Since abortion is a criminal offense in Brazil, embryo reduction is not permitted, even in the case of multiple pregnancies.

Other initiatives for regulating ART in Brazil were undertaken and different bills were proposed – so far unsanctioned – in the National Congress, all of which referred to the first CFM Resolution (Resolution 1385, 1992) as reference.

Feminists and the women's movement did not manage to influence the final format of these bills. As a "scientific-progress-in-itself" discourse prevailed, we may infer that these bills were conceived to protect, first of all, the interests of the medical professionals involved. Indeed, they were proposed by deputies who were also doctors (from different specialties). Currently, the most comprehensive bill is Law 1184 (2013), which incorporated 12 other bills proposed over a decade, but it is still uncertain whether Brazilians will ever have a proper law on ART.

An important landmark was the 1996 Family Planning Law (Law 9263, 1996), prompted by the almost "compulsory" surgical sterilizations widely performed in Brazil, disregarding women's autonomy. This "culture of sterilization" (Berquo, 1993) was debated by activists and socio-demographic authors. As the law states:

> Family Planning is a right of all the citizens and must be granted at the public healthcare level to women, men or couples ... to offer methods for conception or contraception ... Doctors who perform surgical sterilizations but do not report both the procedure and the conditions in which they were undertaken to Sanitary Authorities shall be imprisoned.

For some jurists, most of ART's implications could be regulated and controlled by already existing norms and laws, such as the Family Planning Law[3] and the Civil Code from 2003 (Ciocci, Viana & Borges, 2009; Fachin, 2003). For physicians, having a specific ART law seems to be relevant, as they have been trying hard to influence the legislative process since its onset in the 1990s. The main strategy undertaken by their lobbyists is to claim the difference between a "clinic-of-infertility-for-infertile-couple-in-need-of-a-child", and embryonic stem cell research and other controversial issues later associated with ART, such as same-sex families and commercialization of eggs and wombs (although doctors have always been involved in these practices, for profit or prestige).

But framing ART exclusively as a clinic for infertile couples would become less and less credible, as biotechnology gained considerable strength with the 2005 revision of the Brazilian law on biotechnology (Law 11105, 2005),[4] which includes in its scope stem cell research and circulation of human biological material, reaffirming its non-commercialization. Effectively, in 2004, just before voting began on the new biotech law, CFM issued a particular decision regarding cryopreserved reproductive material, stating that no gamete or embryo could be used in Brazil "if acquired through a commercial transaction, involving foreign countries" (Prata, 2005), as stem cell researchers at universities used to import embryos, mainly from the US.

The new Brazilian biotechnology law (Law 11105, 2005) requirements reinforced monitoring by setting up the SisEmbryo register of frozen embryos, which is operated by the governmental agency Anvisa. But it was only in 2014 that SisEmbryo managed to organize and publish data, self-reported from IVF centers (Table 2.1).[5] No regulation on clinical aspects of ART use came into force, even though the revised biotechnology law explicitly mentions IVF centers as the only source of human embryos, stem cells and reproductive cells for research; spare or non-viable frozen embryos are kept in IVF clinics (Corrêa & Loyola, 2005).

Table 2.1 Total number of embryos donated to embryonic stem cell research in Brazil (2007 to 2013)

Year	Number of donated embryos
2007	643
2008	382
2009	490
2010	748
2011	1,322
2012	315
2013	1,231
Total	**5,131**

Source: SisEmbrio/Anvisa (2014), data obtained on March 27, 2014

The point here is to track frozen embryos, since embryonic stem cell researchers must report to Anvisa which clinics they received biological material from. In fact, in Brazil, semen, embryos or ovarian tissue banks are not separated from clinical practice itself, in banks of tissues and embryos; IVF clinics keep these reproductive materials. The only exception is the recent case of stem cells collected from embryonic cords and placentas, which wealthy families may afford to cryopreserve in certain private laboratories.

In the early 2000s, pressures coming from the international medical field itself, voicing criticisms on risks and undesired effects associated with hormone use and ART procedures, especially concerning multiple pregnancies (WHO, 2002), pushed forward the monitoring of these practices in Brazil and Latin America. RedLara (*Rede Latino-americana de reprodução assistida,* Latin America Assisted Reproduction Network), a regional professional society, improved available data by cataloguing collected records from IVF centers from affiliated clinics, on a voluntary basis. Since 2000 RedLara has also undertaken broader and more complex activities: from accreditation of clinics to logistic support, training and even research on the region (see www.redlara.com).[6]

These reports have provided more accurate information on results and the characteristics of drug use, pregnancies, deliveries, newborns, and different ARTs in Brazil and Latin America. There might still be under-notification, as some IVF centers are not accredited; a considerable problem, involving risks and undesired ART effects that are not being monitored. Brazil has been the country in the region that provides the most data – 50% of all IVF cycles (absolute numbers), in spite of under-notification. Regarding the density of ART usage (relative numbers), Argentina appears to be the country with more procedures per total population of women of reproductive age. Table 2.2 shows the overall results of ART procedures in the region for 2011 (RedLara, 2013).[7]

Table 2.2 ART procedures and access in 2011

Country	Number of clinics	Assisted reproductive techniques					Access***
		IVF*	ICSI*	FET	OD**	Total	
Argentina	25	647	5,398	1,591	2,221	9,857	465
Brazil	54	1,156	12,757	3,745	1,294	18,952	190
Chile	7	161	1,267	325	166	1,919	223
Colombia	9	317	401	127	262	1,107	49
Ecuador	5	79	347	85	159	670	89
Guatemala	1	35	56	8	13	112	16
Mexico	29	1,034	2,349	700	1,185	5,268	91
Nicaragua	1	56	30	0	3	89	31
Panama	1	2	201	31	34	268	156
Peru	5	274	723	148	683	1,828	123
Uruguay	2	14	246	40	58	358	209
Venezuela	6	314	201	109	180	804	121
Total	**145**	**4,089**	**23,976**	**6,909**	**6,258**	**41,232**	**158**

Source: The Latin America Registry, 2011, published in JBRA Assist. Reprod. 17(4), Jul/Aug 2013
*initiated cycles; **includes the transfer of fresh and frozen embryos; ***number of cycles per million women between 15 and 45 years old

One hundred and twenty-eight clinics reported 6,258 oocyte donation (OD) cycles. In 60% of the cases, the purpose was donating, and 40% were egg-sharing practices, i.e. patients undergoing controlled ovarian hyper-stimulation and oocyte pick-up for an autologous treatment, donating part of their gametes to an already known third party.

RedLara (private) and SisEmbrio (public) are becoming sources of information on IVF activities, but according to the opinion of specialists interviewed for this chapter and for previous research, RedLara still have more accurate information than Anvisa on the IVF scenario in Brazil.

Access to ART in Brazil today

ART is neither covered by private health insurance nor widely available, according to the public healthcare system (SUS). Throughout the country, there are very few public services offering the necessary inputs – procedures, drugs, etc. – and those that do understandably have long waiting lists. A recent survey (Souza, 2014) identified 11 public IVF centers in Brazil. Among the 54 centers reported by RedLara for the same period (RedLara, 2013) only one is a public IVF center.

Table 2.3 ART health public services in Brazil. General results from 11 public centers that hold IVF-ICSI and IUI in Brazil – 2013

Public Center	Region	n IUI	n IVF	Source of funds %				Input of Patients %	
				P	R	D	Patients	SUS	Open Access
CEPRA*	MW	21	99	100				100	
HPBSP	SE	11	359	100				100	
UNESP	SE	100	400	70			30		100
USP-SP*	SE	133	324	90			10	100	
USP-RP*	SE	53	447	80			20	100	
ABC-SP	SE	433	1758	2	5	3	90		100
UFRGS*	S	0	240	100				100	
FMG	MW	87	103	100				100	
UFMG*	SE	193	200	80	20			100	
HAA-RJ	SE	0	114	100				30	70
IG-UFRJ	SE	57	0	100					

SE Southest; S South; MW middle-West
Source of funds: P public; R research; D donations; patients – direct payment
*Qualified with extra funds by SUS (Sistema Único de Saúde) – Brasil
USP-RP and CEPRA are accredited RedLara Centers
Open Access means a medical referral is not necessary

Still, there are 120 to 200 clinics, according to Brazilian specialists' estimations. Centers are run by SUS, albeit with very limited options, many difficulties and particular access conditions (see Table 2.1), therefore: "[it] certainly exposes low income people to either unclear or unfair situations of gamete donation and surrogacy" (op. cit., p 47).

As late as 2005, the Ministry of Health ordinance "Policy of Integral ART Care" (*Política de atenção integral à reprodução humana assistida*) is very thorough regarding the investigation of couples, use of drugs, accreditation of medical public services, etc. The ordinance targeted mainly infertile couples and "HIV discordant couples", a policy that was swiftly revoked. SUS now offer mostly diagnostic investigation, possible surgical correction and treatment of sub-fertility in human reproduction services or general hospitals.

In short, access to ART in Brazil is a matter of income or economic power. Additionally, courts have been receiving individual lawsuits demanding access to healthcare and pharmaceuticals, evoking the constitutional principle of the universal right to health. Jurisprudence from the Rio de Janeiro State Court of Justice is quite divergent: some decisions deny the request for State provision of drugs and IVF procedures, claiming their high costs would impact expenses on other diseases affecting a greater number of people; other decisions, also denying the requests, distinguish family planning from the right to health, stating that infertility does not threaten life or health; finally, only one judge, based on a CFM understanding, affirmed that infertility is a pathology and recognized the right to access IVF medicine as a means to enforce the rights to health, life, family and even the right to be happy. The judge also claimed that the State cannot act upon one aspect of family planning (contraception) and be silent on the other (conception).[8]

This unavailability of IVF in any public or refundable private healthcare system leads to proposals that challenge women's reproductive rights and health in Brazil, since they prompt a fertility industry – the commercialization and commodification of women's bodies – in a pattern that is mostly found in low- and middle-income countries (Klein, 2008; SAMA, 2010).

ART access to whom?

The first case study of non-regulated commercialization of ART presented here is the *Programa Acesso*. Set up in 2005 and sponsored by a multinational pharmaceutical firm, Merck, its aims are providing discounted drugs for patients presenting "impaired conception". Beneficiaries not only may "have access" to the company's drugs, but also buy them at cheaper prices. The Access Program operates in association with IVF clinics previously accredited by the company itself.

To enroll in the Access Program, people may visit the website http://www.ism. net.br/programa-acesso/ ("I want to have a baby"), fill in a form with personal and financial data and choose an accredited doctor. Alternatively, accredited clinics may propose enrollment directly to their clients in consultations. Merck has the final word on whether a person is eligible. The eligibility criteria are basically economical: a beneficiary may not be too poor or too rich, but must have enough money to afford drugs and consume services. It is a strategy to enlarge the reproductive medical and pharmaceutical market, whereas the application of these techniques is almost absent in public healthcare in Brazil, and very expensive, severely limiting the pool of potential consumers.

In fact, the Access Program is a branch of a bigger initiative of pharmaceutical companies called Vidalink, which "includes drugs from top pharmaceutical manufacturers such as Altana, Merck, Bayer, Novartis, Biosintética, Organon, Boehringer, Pfizer, Eurofarma, Schering-Plough, Farmoquímica, Stiefel Jannssen-Cilag, Torrent, Eli Lilly Wyeth" (http://www.vidalink.com). Based on a US Pharmacy Benefits Management Model (PBMM), Vidalink claims to have adapted to "the needs of the Brazilian healthcare sector", their objectives being:

> significant cost reduction for end users and for health benefit sponsors; improved access and adherence to treatment; reduction in the risk of self-medication; increased awareness of the correct use of prescription drugs.

As one can read at Vidalink's website (op. cit.): "our mission is to improve the quality of healthcare while providing solutions ... that enhance the bottom line for our clients, which include providers, payers, and suppliers." Vidalink's founders identified Brazil as the largest potential PBM market outside of the United States, based on the fact that the country has the second-largest private healthcare market in the world. They claim to have their own "eligibility platform, encouraging members to adhere and receive discounted prescription services through the Vidalink retail pharmacy network".

This is very controversial, especially considering the principles of SUS' universal public healthcare system in Brazil. Even with all the difficulties faced by SUS, the main orientation for Brazilian public health policies is to expand healthcare coverage in all fields of medicine, and in the most inclusive way. Today, almost 70% of the Brazilian population relies entirely on SUS. A small part of those might be able to access IVF in a subsidized Access Program, but undoubtedly the constitutional individual right to health, the principle of universal access to treatment of SUS and the real needs of Brazilians are being denied.

Since we are yet to find scientific publications on this matter, many questions remain unanswered, particularly regarding the position of other public institutions for the control of diseases and healthcare regulation.

The second case of "hidden" commercialization is the practice of egg sharing or sharing of oocytes in return for financing fertility treatments, undertaken in Brazil since 1994 (Brandi et al., 1995). The real magnitude of this practice is unknown, and many data inconsistencies are expected, since its legitimacy in Brazil is not clear. The Federal Constitution, biotechnology law, the law of transplant and other norms (e.g. CFM Resolution 1392 – Federal Council of Medicine, 1992) reaffirm the non-commercialization of cells, tissues or parts of the human body. Publications by Brazilian specialists in the late 2000s refer to more than ten years of sharing OD Programs (Cavalcante et al., 2005; Lopes, 2008, 2009; Machado et al., 2009; Parames et al., 2014). Would there be financial transactions in oocyte sharing in return for fertility payment?

For some bioethicists, the sharing of oocytes would be more ethical than single OD, since, assuming an interest in treatment from both recipient and donor, the latter would only be under risk (use of drugs, procedures) with an expected benefit in return. This takes us back to the framing of donation when it comes to reproductive matters: would it be altruistic, familial or commercial? In countries such as Brazil, where there is no compensation for donation and it is a criminal offense to profit from selling human cells and tissues, the altruistic perspective prevails.

For those supporting it, egg sharing in return for financial support for treatment would involve a system of need-adjusted reciprocity, ethically "better" than paying for oocytes (Kahan, 2009), even if it involves egg sharing between women from two countries with very different socio-economic realities (Heng, 2005).

In some countries, to maximize the number of retrievable oocytes, prospective egg-sharers are often restricted to younger women with indications for either male-factor or mild female-factor sub-fertility. Which doses of gonadotropins are to be given to the donor in egg sharing? Is it necessary and ethically acceptable to subject younger women with good prognosis to high dosages of hormones, just for the sake of maximizing the yield of retrievable oocytes for egg sharing or even selling? Regarding the number of fertilized oocytes picked up vs embryos transferred, the question is how to assess the chances for two women with different ages. Even the cost of treatment, which in Brazil is paid in full by the patients, is discussed.

In Brazil, we can propose, egg sharing has a standard: women from different socioeconomic strata frequently engage in donor and recipient roles, since 95% of complex procedures are found only in private healthcare and are therefore inaccessible to most people, who cannot afford ART procedures and medicine at all. In such a context, there is no choice. The "Brazilian model" involves a younger woman with tube diseases (often as a secondary result from repeated STD or clandestine and badly performed abortions), but who has oocytes. She can be recruited in public hospitals, from their infertility ward or even their emergency room.[9] At the other end, there is an older woman with hormonal impairment, who will pay for the two treatments, her own and the donor's. Doctors working in both medical sectors provide the link and acquire two patients. In ethical terms, it is very difficult to ensure transparency and avoid undue inducement in the procurement of shared donor oocytes. How can donation be separated from the exploitation of childless poorer women? Would they still be donors if ART were available in public healthcare? Additionally, some technical aspects may not be ignored, such as women's age, which is the key aspect to success rates (Corrêa, 2000).

Moreover, there are also the ethically questionable surrogacy websites, such as www.surrogatefinder.com,[10] that connect donors and recipients in exclusively commercial transactions that take place mostly across borders.

Final considerations

The two cases brought up in this chapter depict the paradoxical way ART entered and was established in Brazil, mainly in private healthcare, as a profitable practice.

The Brazilian reproductive health scenario shows detrimental conditions for fertility and conception: there is a high prevalence of sexually transmitted diseases, not controlled, that can lead to secondary infertilities; abortion is still a crime but has been performed clandestinely on a wide scale as a radical contraceptive method used in extreme conditions – most cases involving poor women under hazardous conditions (Diniz & Correa, 2009); over 50% of deliveries are C-sections during which surgical sterilizations are performed. The offer of contraceptive reversible methods should imply a more efficient reproductive health service, which, however, is not always available around Brazil. These detrimental situations to conception and fertility are the result of precarious family planning services. Despite the accumulation of advanced knowledge and technology, mediocre rates in women's health still persist. But the groups of females going through these processes of exclusion to medical practices are not the same groups who decide to go through ART in Brazil, in the private sector of medicine.

In spite of the sanitary, ethical and legal controversies that underlie the application of ART and its outcomes, the social values attached to family, domestic life, maternity and personal achievement through parenthood deem the desire for having children socially legitimate, and justify the search for accessing these techniques "at any cost".

In commercial arrangements, such as egg-sharing programs in return for financing fertility treatment, there is both the reinforcement of those more or less traditional values as well as the production of disorder, domination and even exploitation of women (North–South reproductive tourism). These practices also lead to institutional disarrangements, considering the tensions between the legal framework of Brazil's universal public healthcare system (SUS) and the almost complete lack of ART in public healthcare, in low- and middle-income countries.

There is no doubt that the policies (as well as the lack of policies, for that matter) become, in this sense, biopolitics, as indicated by ART results and implications that have been transforming not only the biological order, but also the social one. Thus, as scientists, researchers and activists, we may ask ourselves how we can intervene in these processes of biological and social reorganization in the field of reproduction, produced by the unequal availability and access to public healthcare services of ART, along with its dissemination around the globe, worsening the North–South imbalance and making room for unfair and ethically questionable practices.

Notes

1 Soap Operas: "*Belly for Hire*" (1991) and "*The Clone*" (2001).
2 SUS was not conceived for the poor. Approximately 70% of Brazilians rely only on public healthcare. Around 30% also have private health insurance that constitutes the so-called supplementary healthcare (*saúde suplementar*). The wealthiest 1% of citizens opt not to have private insurance as they can afford to directly purchase healthcare in private medicine (these are the group that have access to ART).
3 Brasil Código Civil Brasileiro Subtítulo II Das Relações de Parentesco (art 1591 a 1597) in force since 2003.
4 Ministério da Saúde Portaria/GM 426/ 22 de março 2005. Política Nacional de Atenção Integral à Reprodução Humana Assistida 2005.

5 For SISEMBRIO: http://portal.anvisa.gov.br/wps/wcm/connect/15ecee804745885f91
   e1d53fbc4c6735/relatorio_sisembrio.pdf
6 The *Jornal Brasileiro de Reprodução Assistida*, official publication of the Brazilian Society
   for Assisted Reproduction (SBRA), also publishes data from the annual RedLara report.
7 The 2011 Latin America Registry report a total of 41,223 cycles. From this total, 4,089
   were IVF cycles and 23,976 ICSI; 6,909 involved frozen embryo transfer and 6,258
   oocytes donation (OD). We observe a progressive increase of micromanipulations
   techniques (ICSI), a still more invasive procedure than IVF; the majority of cases being
   related to male factor fertility impairments. Multiple pregnancies are still high. (IFFS,
   2013; Zegers-Hochschild, 2013; Souza, 2014).
8 http://www.tjrj.jus.br/documents/10136/1019732/fertilizacao-in-vitro.pdf (Retrieved 1
   October, 2014) I thank my doctorate student Koichi Kameda, who has a background in
   Law studies and helped me to gather these data.
9 Previously, another group of specialists proposed collecting oocytes during pelvic
   surgical interventions (Donadio, 1999).
10 For instance, www.surrogatefinder.com/surrogates/5208/; www.premiereggdonors.
   com/south-american-egg-donors/www.eggdonor4u.com. In the last one, we read: "Are
   you looking for an egg donor who is located in Brazil, Argentina or South America?
   We have a large international database of egg donors... and we see the faces of women
   offering their services."

References

Becker G & Nachtigall RD. 1992. Eager for medicalization: the social production of infertility as a disease. *Sociology of Health and Illness,* 14(4):456–471.
Berquo E. 1993. Brasil um caso exemplar – anticoncepção e partos cirúrgicos – à espera de uma ação exemplar. *Estudos Feministas,* 1(2).
Brandi MC, Costa RR, Lopes JRC, Nogueira TML, Barbosa AH, Nakagawa HM, Medina-Lopes MDD, Costa TBM, Tenório MC, Souza RC; Benedetti AR, de Melo, ML. 1995. Doação compartilhada de óvulos (DOC). *Reprodução e Climatério,* 10:148–150.
Cavalcante E, Juliano Y, Pereira DM, Catafestall E, Shimabukuroll L, Curyll MCFDS, Cavagna M. 2005. Resultados das técnicas de reprodução assistida em mulheres doadoras de oócitos no ciclo de tratamento. *Rev Bras. Ginecol Obstet,* 27(11):661–664.
Ciocci D, Viana RGC, Borges Jr E. 2009. Aspectos legais na utilização de gametas e embriões nas técnicas de reprodução humana assistida. *JBRA Assist Reprod,* July/ August/ September 13(3).
Federal Council of Medicine (Conselho Federal de Medicina, CFM). 1992. Resolução 1358. Normas éticas para a utilização das técnicas de reprodução assistida. Revised in 2010; Revised in 2013.
Corea G. 1985. *The Mother Machine. Reproductive Technologies from Artificial Insemination to Artificial Wombs.* New York: Harper&Row.
Corrêa MCDV & Loyola MA. 2005. Reprodução e Bioética. A regulação da reprodução assistida no Brasil. *Cadernos CRH* Salvador, 18(33):103–112.
Corrêa MCDV. 1997. A tecnologia a serviço de um sonho. Um estudo sobre a reprodução assistida no Brasil [Tese de Doutorado]. Rio de Janeiro: Instituto de Medicina Social.
Corrêa MCDV. 2000. Novas tecnologias reprodutivas: doação de óvulos. O que pode ser novo nesse campo? [New reproductive technologies: oocyte donation. What could be new in this field?] *Cad. Saúde Pública,* Rio de Janeiro July/Sept, 16(3):863–870.
Diniz D, Corrêa M, Squinca F, Braga K. 2009. Abortion: 20 years of Brazilian research. *Cad. Saúde Pública,* Rio de Janeiro Apr. 25(4)939–942.

Donadio N. 1999. Óvulo doações por mulheres de 36 anos e férteis com proles definidas durante pequenas cirurgias laparoscópicas. *Jornal Brasileiro de Reprodução Assistida*, 3: http://www.sbra.com.br

Fachin LEA. 2003. *Nova Filiação: o biodireito e as relações parentais: o estabelecimento da paternidade-fi liação e os efeitos jurídicos da reprodução assistida heteróloga*. Rio de Janeiro: Renovar.

Franco Jr. JGE & Wheba S. 1994. I Registro Brasileiro sobre o uso das técnicas de reprodução assistida. *Reprodução*, 9(3).

Heng BH. 2005. Ethics, social legal, counseling: International egg-sharing to provide donor oocytes for clinical assisted reproduction and derivation of nuclear transfer stem cells. *RBM* October 2005, II(6):676–678.

IFFS (International Federation of Fertility Societies). 2013. SJ Ory & P Devroye (eds). Surveillance. Available at: https://c.ymcdn.com/sites/iffs.site-ym.com/resource/resmgr/ iffs_surveillance_09-19-13.pdf

Kahan SK. 2009. Incentivizing organ donation: a proposal to end the organ shortage. *Hofstra Law Review*, 38(2):757–791.

Klein R. 2008. From test-tube women to bodies without women. *Women's Studies International Forum*, 31:157–175.

Lopes JRC. 2008. A idade da receptora influencia os resultados de gravidez clinica em um Programa de Doação Compartilhada de Ovulos (DOC) JBRA – *Jornal Brasileiro de Reprodução Assistida*, 13(1).

Lopes JRC. 2009. Ovo recepção perfil das pacientes em lista de espera no programa do Hospital Regional da Asa Sul, Brasilia. *Rev Bras. Ginecol Obstet*, 29(9):459–464.

Machado CE, Sutter C, Costa ALE. 2009. Recepção de óvulos doados: a alternativa para a maternidade tardia. *JBRA – Jornal Brasileiro de Reprodução Assistida*, 13(4).

Parames, SFFLS & Almada-Colucci J. 2014. What influences oocyte donation when there is no financial compensation? *Repodução e Climatério*, 29(1):8–12.

Prata H. 2005. Regulation of Assisted Reproductive Techniques. *JIBL*, 02:71–75.

RedLara. 2013. The Latin America Registry, 2011, in *JBRA Assisted Reproduction*, Jul/ Aug 17(4).

Reis Ana RG. 1987. IVF in Brazil: The Story Told By the Newspapers, in *Made to Order: The Myth of Reproductive and Genetic Progress*, Spallone P & Steinberg Deborah L (eds). Oxford: Pergamon Press.

SAMA (The Resource Group for Women and Health). 2010. *Unravelling the fertility industry: challenges and strategies for movement building*. International Consultation on Commercial, Economic and Ethical and Aspects of Assisted Reproductive Technologies. A report, January 22–24, 2010.

Souza MCB. 2014. Latin America and access to Assisted Reproductive Techniques: a Brazilian Perspective. *JBRA Assisted Reproduction*, 18(2):47–51.

WHO (World Health Organization). 2002. *Current practices and controversies in assisted reproduction report of a meeting*, in Vayena, Rowe, Griffin (eds). Geneva: Report of a WHO meeting on "Medical, Ethical and Social Aspects of Assisted Reproduction".

Zegers-Hochschild F, Adamson GD, de Mouzon J, Ishihara O, Mansour R, Nygren K, Sullivan E, Vanderpoel S. 2013. International Committee for Monitoring Assisted Reproductive Technology (ICMART) and the World Health Organization (WHO) revised glossary of ART technology. *Fertility and Sterility*, 92(5).

3   The gendered nature of infertility and ARTs

Sarojini Nadimpally & Vrinda Marwah

Introduction

Within India's growing medical market and medical tourism industry, ARTs have been added to the long list of cheap and high-tech services the country is selling to the world. Estimates suggest that the total market size of the fertility industry in India is INR 1700 crore (approx. USD 276 million) and is expected to reach INR 14,000 crore (approx. USD 2.2 billion) in the next 10 years, growing at 24% annually. The phenomenal growth of ARTs in India has been enabled by the economic climate of the country's post-liberalisation era, which led to an exponential growth in its private medical sector. ARTs are predominantly part of this private medical market. Today the public health system in India – itself in a state of serious neglect – does not offer even basic preventive, curative and counselling services for infertility, but the country is being pegged as a global 'reproductive tourism' destination (Reddy and Qadeer 2010). ARTs are offered in India to whoever can pay, from India or abroad. While there are instances of lower income families incurring disproportionately huge expenditure – by selling off their assets, for example – in the hope of having a biologically related child, within India the cost of ARTs means it is predominantly accessible only to the privileged upper and middle classes. To the world, India offers the comparative advantage of medical and technological expertise at relatively lower costs, with English-speaking staff, world-famous tourist destinations, and an unregulated environment. Crucially, India also has an ample supply of poor women willing to be egg donors and surrogates. No regulation exists for the industry, except for a set of non-binding guidelines by the Indian Council of Medical Research (ICMR 2005), and a proposed law in draft form which has gone through multiple revisions but is yet to be tabled before parliament (ICMR 2010).

In the absence of reliable national statistics, ART registries, or monitoring bodies that can give an overview of ARTs or surrogacy in India, most of the information about the women users of ARTs is anecdotal. Regardless, the wider patriarchal association of woman-as-body is a long continuing one, and the use and abuse of women's bodies in other contexts has been written about extensively (Das 1986; Chatterjee 1989; Uberoi 1990). Women's bodies are signs through which men communicate with each other; at the level of community and nation, women are held up as signifiers and repositories of honour, and at more individual levels, notions of good and bad behaviour constantly mediate the relationship women have with their bodies. To 'behave like a good woman', then, is to deploy and enact the body in ways that win patriarchal favour, and to be a 'misbehaving' woman/body is, inversely, to excite patriarchal disfavour through non-conformism, or even wilful defiance.

This chapter explores the construction of womanhood-as-motherhood, such that non-conforming bodies of childless and/or infertile women are seen as gender non-performers, as not keeping their side of the 'gender bargain'. Such logic sets the tone for the mistreatment of childless and/or infertile women, who are blamed for their 'lack'. In accessing ARTs, it is this lack that is sought to be corrected. The process of treatment that follows continues to be over-determined by gender. That women bear the burden of (in)fertility is clear even in cases of male factor infertility, and through their anxiety about treatment, lack of coping mechanisms during treatment, and lack of control over treatment. This essay also examines how sex and sexuality get constructed through ARTs – first, at the level of discourse, as being in need of control, and then at the level of treatment, through regulation and medicalisation. We find, however, that while gender organises experience, experience remains also individual, and far from homogenous.

Methodology

This paper draws from the research *Constructing Conceptions: The Mapping of Assisted Reproductive Technologies in India*,[1] conducted by SAMA, a Delhi-based resource group working on issues at the intersection of gender and health. This research was conducted from 2008 to 2010 in the three states of Uttar Pradesh (UP), Orissa (OR), and Tamil Nadu (TN) in India, with the objective of understanding the economic and commercial aspects of ART provision and proliferation, as well as access to and implications of these technologies in the Indian context. As part of the research, 43 ART providers and 86 female users, who were undergoing intra uterine insemination (IUI), in vitro fertilisation (IVF), or intra cytoplasmic sperm injection (ICSI), were recruited from ART clinics and interviewed. The design of the research was essentially exploratory and qualitative, and sought to document experiences and draw general conclusions based on analyses. The mode of primary data collection involved in-depth interviews, participant observation, and focus group discussions. A review of secondary literature, including of promotional materials of clinics, was also undertaken. A team of advisors was instituted to oversee the ethical and methodological aspects of the research. While selecting research sites, a deliberate attempt was made to choose a sample that contained diverse geographical areas with diverse human development indicators, representing different stages of the development of the ART industry in India. As such, the selection of states was purposive, with ARTs in Tamil Nadu being the most commercial and Orissa being the least. ART providers identified through a mapping exercise were approached directly, and women users were approached through clinics. All names have been codified to maintain anonymity; the names of users (U) and providers (P) have been documented with initials of the state coming first in the codes given. The research employs the word 'user' rather than 'patient' because ARTs circumvent infertility rather than cure it. The term ART 'provider' is used because it refers to doctors, embryologists, counsellors, etc., i.e. all categories of personnel involved in the provision of ARTs, including but not limited to medical doctors.

The research sample consisted of users from different castes and religions (overwhelmingly Hindu), all of whom were married. However, this should not indicate that the market is blind to caste and religion, or that it bears the potential to liberate us from ascriptive identities. Rather, access to ARTs is mediated by identities of gender, sexuality, caste, religion, class, etc. In India, given that caste is classed, access to ARTs must be understood as being mediated most significantly by class, and therefore by caste. Similarly, religion can be understood as often circumscribing the limits of technology use, as much as technology is deployed in ways that preserve and perpetuate religious affiliations. For instance, advice on the 'permissibility' of ARTs, particularly in the case of use of donor gametes, may be sought from a local religious leader, just as a gamete donor from a particular religion may be sought over others. While data on monthly income was sought from users, it did not give a clear picture of the distribution of data by class.

This research highlighted some key features of India's ART industry, which is attracting clientele through aggressive marketing and reducing operational costs through schemes, treatment in camps and batches. In the absence of regulation, there is a lack of standardisation in terms of costs, procedures, information, counselling, and consent. Additionally, there is potential for unethical practices like sex selection and multiple-embryo implantation that threaten women's health and rights. The ART industry also deploys and (re)produces the patriarchal imperative to mother, while being able to posit and market itself as pro-women, 'delivering desperate women' from the 'trauma' of 'childlessness'.

The woman-as-mother: fertility as a social imperative

Gender in India is constituted through the demonstration that one is capable of certain transactions, which frame both gender and sexuality as specifically social performances. To be a woman or a man is to bear the potential to perform and fulfil socially prescribed roles for a woman or a man. Particularly, to be a woman is to perform the mother role. Inversely, the non-performance of gender is seen as meriting *social intervention*. The absence of offspring in a marriage becomes more visible than their presence (Khanna 2006: 16; Bharadwaj 2003).

> When couples don't have children, elders don't leave it alone. They put a lot of pressure to go in for check-ups, treatments etc. Because of the pressure, couples tend to think that it is essential for them to have their own child. We start thinking about the future. Even if we have not been thinking about this, they make us think about it.
>
> TNU-10

These non-performing bodies of the childless/infertile are seen as exceptions to and distortions of the category of woman, to be corrected and restored, rather than as evidence of the uninhabitability and instability of the category itself. Childlessness evokes multiple stigmas and exclusions from social, even familial life, for which women predominantly carry the burden (Jejeebhoy 1998). Actual and anticipated rude comments at social functions force many women to become social recluses (Unisa 1999), and within the family, childless women find their position as married women threatened (Prakasamma 1999).

> Everyone else in the family would be invited for some function or the other, but not me. When this happened a few times, I decided I will stop going myself.
>
> UPU-4

Women's anxiety about motherhood was deeply internalised, even in instances where their families and communities were supportive of them, or where it was clear that the 'problem' was not with them.

> Women mostly think even before any tests are done that they are the ones with the problem. We have to really insist on the husband getting tested as well.
>
> TNP-5

Women with supportive husbands categorically stated that 'even though' the problem was with them, their husbands 'still' loved them, thus betraying the feeling that they could not expect love and support from their husbands as a matter of course. It qualified rather, as an 'in spite of'; an extraordinary response to an extraordinary situation. Many women themselves ask their husbands to remarry, especially (though not only) when they discover that the 'problem' is with them. On the other hand, in only one user interview, the husband insisted that his wife marry again. Instances of providers blaming the woman for her infertility, at least in part, were also many. Delayed fertility was an oft-cited reason for female factor infertility.

> Yes definitely, women want to be financially independent and have their own standing, and are getting very serious about their careers. At the same time, we are also becoming very westernised – women are realising that they enjoy being single, not being answerable to anyone. They are also enjoying their sex lives before marriage. So all said and done, women are definitely delaying their marriages.
>
> TNP-8

These comments reveal an anxiety about the status of marriage and its progression to biological reproduction, perceived to be under threat from women's mobility, professional agency, and their 'new-age' re-prioritisation, whether real or imagined. The providers prescribe the 'ideal' age for marriage, so as to capitalise on women's 'optimum' eggs and their 'appropriate' fertility window, indicating that women are responsible for how their bodies 'behave'. It becomes clear, therefore, that the equation of womanhood with motherhood is not just socially prescribed, but like all apparently 'natural' roles, is also socially regulated. Through motherhood a woman gains social legitimacy as a 'complete' or 'true' woman.

Table 3.1 Income profile of the users

Income range (INR) per month	Rural			Semi-urban			Urban			Total
	OR	UP	TN	OR	UP	TN	OR	UP	TN	
2,000–4,000	4	–	1	–	–	1	1	–	4	11
4,001–10,000	6	–	4	1		1	2	2	7	23
10,001–20,000	6	–	1	3	–	2	–	1	6	19
20,001–50,000	–	–	–	1	–	2	2	3	6	14
50,001–1,000,000	1	–	1	–	1	–	–	–	2	5
1,00,001–5,000,000	–	–	–	–	1	–	–	1	–	2
Did not give/not available	2	1	–	–	2	1	1	1	4*	12
Total	19	1	7	5	4	7	6	8	29	86

* Three of these were family incomes and hence respondents were unable to give an amount.
Source: Constructing Conceptions, SAMA 2010

Non-man: male factor infertility and its effects on women

> In almost all cases of a couple not being able to have a child, it is the woman who is generally tortured. Even in cases of male infertility in a couple, it is the woman who is tortured and goes through the entire mental trauma. Eventually only women are treated for any kind of infertility problem, even when male factor infertility is involved. Women undergo the tests and treatment. Men are not even ready to undergo a simple semen analysis test. They always feel that there can be no problem with them. The male ego is such that they won't tolerate any questioning of their masculinity and capacity to father a child...
>
> ORU-1

Not surprisingly, women were blamed even in cases of male factor infertility. The threat of abandonment, divorce, or polygamy was faced by women respondents more commonly, even in cases where the diagnosis was unclear or confirmed male factor infertility. This sense of marital insecurity is a profoundly gendered experience, with no threats of remarriage being made by the interviewed women to their husbands. Some women made it clear that they would rather bear the burden of infertility than disclose a diagnosis of male factor infertility.

> The standard question is, 'Have you got a child; why the delay?' I cannot tell anyone that the problem is with my husband because people will say all kinds of things for male factor infertility. He will lose respect in society. They call

men '*potta*' (effeminate). I cannot tolerate all this and I remain silent when people ask me about a child.

TNU-3

In a particularly stark instance, TNU-29's in-laws could not come to terms with their son's diagnosis of azoospermia and were being hostile to the couple; they had started cooking separately and stopped talking to their son completely. Nonetheless, they did not give their relatives the real picture of the couple's infertility, and the relatives continued to think the 'problem' was with the wife. Many providers too confirmed that people found a diagnosis of male factor infertility difficult to reconcile with.

> We get a number of requests from husbands who have defective semen sample to not divulge details to their family members or their wives. They don't even want to let the wife know! The wife who gets abused every day because of this! There was a case where the husband's sperm was not up to the mark. The mother-in-law came up to me and said that first of all I should not tell the wife, because she will not respect her son! Then she said that we should use the father-in-law's sperm in place of the husband's. It was so unbelievable.

UPP-22

Some providers suggested that the attitude of men towards infertility was shifting, and that there were also some men diagnosed with male factor infertility who were sensitive towards their wives. However, many men were either in denial or were resisting treatment for male factor infertility. At a societal level, while a misbehaving female body is highly visible and subject to various forms of social control, a misbehaving male body is shrouded in secrecy and its reputation is sought to be protected from 'being called effeminate or lacking', 'losing respect', or 'psychological' harm. The association of masculinity with virility and strength is integral to gender norms, just as the performance of motherhood is to femininity.

Treatment: access, control, and coping mechanisms

Women accessing infertility treatments experience feelings of not 'trying hard enough' in their efforts to be 'woman enough'. This is demonstrated in feelings of tension and anxiety throughout the course of a treatment that is pursued quite relentlessly, sometimes until the couple can no longer afford a satisfactory standard of living, and sometimes even beyond that. These feelings go beyond routine treatment response; they appear as symptoms of anxiety about a gender disruption that refuses to get treated. Further, since infertility treatment aims to set right gender deviance or non-performance by completing an incomplete family, it is seldom recognised as being incapable of completion. Couples often push for, and are pushed into, more and more treatments. Concerns have been raised about the self-perpetuating nature of ART treatments, with doctors now debating the point at which, if at all, couples should be advised to stop treatment (Brakman and Scholz 2006: 63).

> We have decided not to go for any other treatment. I think it is beyond us now. We are not even in a position to maintain a decent life for ourselves. We have to compromise on many aspects. We cannot eat the way we want. Even the kinds of clothes we wear are not what we would like. Now it is completely out of the question to go for treatment again. Sometimes I feel that I will go mad by thinking about all these things.
>
> ORU-7

Couples employ different coping mechanisms in response to a felt lack of control over their circumstances. However, whether and what methods were available to individuals to cope seemed contingent on gender. For instance, ORU-3's husband had been taking courses on the 'art of living' which were helping him maintain a 'positive frame of mind'. Since most of the men were working outside of the home, they were able to occupy and distract themselves in ways that women who stayed at home could not. Both the men and the women acknowledged this difference. Women also lack temporary exit options that are available to men.

> When I feel very bad, I go to the bathroom and cry. I immerse myself in house work. When I did not conceive after the first IVF, my husband got depressed, so he did not come home for three–four days. Some nights he stays out drinking with friends and does not come home.
>
> ORU-28

Many women reported experiencing feelings of dejection, desperation, and isolation. ORU-22 would cry to herself and wonder why this has happened to her. The personal imaginary of infertility seems disproportionately affected by gender. Women appear to be more likely and used to taking the 'blame' and despairing over 'why me'.

Other than a couple of stray instances, the research also makes evident the mostly male control over the use of ARTs. Wives are often largely unaware of their medical diagnosis, and are unable to exert much control over the course, length, and type of infertility treatment they are subjected to. While often both the husband and the wife are unaware of their exact diagnosis and the details of their treatment, the wife is almost always much less informed than her husband, including when the treatment is for female factor infertility.

> Whatever the information, it was given to my husband (by the doctor). Wherever he says to go (for treatment), I go, whether I want to or not.
>
> ORU-17

In so many years, I realise that the status of women has not changed much, regardless of how educated or qualified they may be. Men feel that if there is a problem with women, they should just be put aside and men should remarry. They are reluctant to spend money on treatment for women if there is a problem, even if it is minor and can be easily treated.

TNP-19

Many accounts revealed the difficulties that women face in accessing healthcare. ORU-29 would fight with her husband to be taken to a doctor, but he would refuse. Then she decided to go with her father. However, the doctor sent her back, insisting that she come with her husband instead.

In some cases, no matter the diagnosis, the wife's parents were paying, at least in part, for the couple's treatment, revealing that the responsibility for fertility is seen to lie with the woman, and by extension, her parents and family.

Usually parents of the girl bring her (for treatment), even in the first instance, as though they are responsible for some "defective" goods.

TNP-19

In addition to ARTs, many users sought infertility treatments that were outside the allopathic model itself. Treatment trajectories of users revealed long and complex journeys, involving methods as diverse as alternative therapies of unani, ayurveda, homeopathy, as well as religious ritualism and worship.

I had an allergy due to the Siddha medicines. I feel sick after having all kinds of medicines. My body was punctured three times for laparoscopy. I digested everything for the sake of my child. I feel that my body was used as an experiment for all kinds of treatment.

TNU-17

This interplay of what lies 'inside' the ART clinic as well as what lies 'outside' had the potential to render couples, and particularly women, doubly vulnerable to the negative effects of allopathic and non-allopathic treatment methods.

Sexuality and ARTs

The absence of any institutionalised sex education curricula (re)produces the silence around sexuality, as well as an utter lack of awareness about the fertility cycle. This contributes to infertility, real and perceived, and consequently to many unnecessary treatments for preventable conditions.

Lack of sex education is a major factor for non-conception ... In our society, sex is still a very taboo topic and parents do not talk about this openly with their children. When these children grow up, they don't have adequate knowledge about sexual issues ... There is no awareness about the woman's reproductive cycle.

ORU-1

Some comments by providers revealed a great deal of anxiety about sex and sexuality today, particularly with regard to women.

Nowadays infertility is increasing because there is more sexual freedom and later in life, a heavy price has to be paid for it.

TNP-3

Left and right use of contraceptives, premarital sex, early sex, and then unsafe abortions are responsible for infertility. During our time in school, we used to have a subject called Moral Science. We were taught that our body is a temple and we should keep it as pure as possible. Love and respect your body and soul. Sex should not be as common as food. There is a difference between animal and man, and this is it. Even our Vedas say the same thing ... The same act which is wrong before marriage becomes right after it. And now you have Pill 72, i-Pill, etc., which actually harm women's health. There is an increase in STDs, unwanted pregnancies, incomplete abortions, heavy bleeding, and anaemia. They (women) get D&C (dilation and curettage) done from an unregistered practitioner; tubes blocked, finished; the woman cannot conceive anymore. When women come to us and we find out that they had once conceived and aborted, they request us not to tell their husbands.

UPP-15

This comment is particularly revealing, as it conveys a strong moral-religious discourse around the body's sexuality, which differentiates the 'good' woman from the 'bad'. Female sexuality is considered valid and acceptable only within marriage and sexual pleasure outside marriage is seen as corrupt and dangerous.

Of the couples that chose to comment on their sexual lives, several mentioned that childlessness and ART treatment had made an impact. The treatment process constructed their sexuality as being in need of control. Couples found themselves under a sort of sexual surveillance, and had to have sex according to a 'plan'.

Our sexual life is fine, but now we have sex to conceive. I cannot say that there is pleasure in our sexual life; rather there is pressure to perform better and have a child. Now our sexual life is to have a child.

TNU-13

On the other hand, some couples also denied that their sexual life had been affected by their condition and treatment.

> Our sexual relationship has not been affected in any way. In fact, he *[husband]* has become more caring now. He gives me a lot of attention.
>
> UPU-8

It was clear from the interviews that the lack of sex education was a factor in infertility. However, providers also betrayed a sex-negative attitude that was disapproving of women's sexual freedoms (while men's sexuality was not discussed). The sex lives of couples was also medicalised and monitored closely with the singular aim of conception. How this impacted a couple was variable, with many citing it as a problem and some saying it had no impact on the relationship.

Stigma, discrimination, and violence

The inability to keep one's side of the gender 'bargain' is seen, including by oneself, as justifying loss of privilege, even violence. Often, women did not challenge or question the harassment and violence by their husbands but rather, claimed to 'understand' this behaviour. ORU-9 stated matter-of-factly, 'When outsiders say something, I take out my frustration on her (wife). But that is only for some time.' His wife agreed, 'Definitely, he goes out and if people say something won't he feel bad?' Both insisted that their relationship was not strained.

In an illustration of the classic blaming-the-victim syndrome, women are often considered as having brought on their infertility. Blame can be fixed with the woman through many routes. Interestingly, women reported being taunted in their marital homes because of too much and too little dowry, both of which compounded the stigma they had to face because of infertility. ORU-30's mother-in-law would tell her that she came with a lot of dowry because she is infertile and 'cursed', while ORU-27 insisted that her mother-in-law did not like her because hers was a love marriage with no dowry and now, no child.

UPU-11 was asked by a *baba* (healer) to wash her husband's feet and drink that water on a regular basis, suggesting that she needs to prove her devotion to her husband; perhaps women who cannot conceive are women who are not completely devoted to their husbands? Her sisters-in-law tell her that she doesn't have the qualities of a mother.

> Everyone in the family said I am unfit to beget a child. This statement shattered me. I have cried for many nights and even now, I cannot sleep soundly.
>
> TNU-12

ORU-6 narrated the story of a woman she had met at the infertility clinic whose sister-in-law did not allow her to hang her washed clothes to dry with the rest of the family's. Here the 'perverse' and 'polluted' body was seen as carrying the potential to pervert and pollute other bodies, thus justifying the distancing of the gender non-performers from the gender performers.

> Nobody likes me because I don't have a child. My husband fights with me when I ask him to take me to a doctor … He beats me for the smallest of

reasons … My nieces and nephews don't come near me. If they do, then their mothers don't like it.

ORU-26

Violence forms both the causes and the consequences of infertility. Systemically, the myriad forms of violence – experienced disproportionately by women – are not prioritised by institutions or individuals. For instance, infertility may be a result of occupational health hazards, untreated sexually transmitted infections, or poorly conducted abortions, all of which reflect systemic neglect in the Indian context of a collapsing public health system. On the other end of this spectrum lies violence resulting from infertility, which is highlighted in user interviews. This kind of violence may be physical, sexual, or mental; however, when asked about violence faced due to infertility, women responded with reference to physical violence, while events of mental/emotional violence, though clear from the narratives, were not reported explicitly as violence. However, the trauma that results from mental/emotional violence, though manifested differently, is not *less* than physical violence. In fact, it can be equally fatal, and even more so, as it pushes women to thoughts of suicide.

> There is definitely pressure from everywhere when you are not able to conceive after so many years of marriage. People say harsh things like you are a *banjh* (barren) and one should not see your face … When the doctor said that there is a problem with me, even my own family members started to blame me. Sometimes I used to feel so desperate that I even thought of committing suicide … The problem was with me so what could I do?
>
> ORU-21

Further, a sense of desperation and entrapment is evident as ORU-21 blames herself, and her lack of choice ('… what could I do?'). Juxtaposed against the discourse of 'choice' that is employed by providers to promote treatments, it is interesting to note that what appears to be pushing the infertility business is an utter lack of choice that women feel they have in the event of infertility.

Conclusion

Women, and men, are not homogenous categories. They are differentiated by identities like class, caste, race, etc. that influence their needs and interests, but also by individual characteristics. There is an important distinction between women as a socially subordinate *category* and women as a highly diverse group of *individuals*. As such, different men, women, and couples will experience and act on new technologies for assisting reproduction in ways that reflect 'some combination of their structural positioning and their own unique individual histories' (Kabeer 2001: 20).

Yet, while accounting for individual differences in individuals' experiences, user and provider interviews highlight also how gender operates as both an organising principle and a personal identity. Gender organises the imaginary and real burden of infertility, as well as coping mechanisms and technological fixes for infertility. Interviews reveal not only women's negotiations of the 'interruption' to normative gender performance that is infertility, but rather, the uninhabitable nature of gender itself. In assisting reproduction, this technology is also assisting gender; in making mothers, it is also making women insofar as the non-mother is seen and may see herself as the non-woman.

Moreover, the entire ART enterprise is symptomatic of the 'uncritical acceptance of the biologic paradigm', where *biologic* describes not just genetic/ biological families, but also the bias in favour of such families (Brakman and Scholz 2006: 59). ARTs by their very nature are used when the purely biological/ natural route is unsuccessful. They seek to correct the failure of a pure biologic, and though they are able to ensure only an impure biologic, it is in upholding some semblance of the biologic that their true value lies. The industry is fuelled, then, by the 'imperative that it is better to come as close as possible to biological reproduction' (Brakman and Scholz 2006: 64).

Further, while no such instances were contained in this research sample, the potential in these technologies for the subversion of the heteronormative family through their use by non-normative constituencies such as single women, and lesbian, gay, bisexual, transgender, and queer (LGBTQ) individuals and couples is another gender dimension that merits examination. Overall, the life of these technologies is still unfolding, as are their practical and political implications.

Note

1 The authors would like to acknowledge the entire SAMA team for their contribution to this research. Overall co-ordination of the research was done by Nadimpally Sarojini, and state level co-ordination was by Deepa Venkatachalam, Preeti Nayak, Anjali Shenoi, Vrinda Marwah, and Aastha Sharma, with research assistance from Susheela Singh, N. Srilakshmi, Truptimayee Rout, Beenu Rawat, Saalai Selvam, and Bhawna Rawat. Valuable inputs were given by Manjeer Mukherjee and Padmini Swaminathan. The research was supported by IDRC India.

References

Bharadwaj, A. (2003). Why Adoption is not an Option in India: the Visibility of Infertility, the Secrecy of Donor Insemination, and other Cultural Complexities. *Social Science & Medicine*, 56(9):1867–1880.
Brakman, S.V. & Scholz, S.J. (2006). Adoption, ART, and a Re-Conception of the Maternal Body: Toward Embodied Maternity. *Hypatia*, 21(1):54–73.
Chatterjee, P. (1989). Colonialism, Nationalism, and Colonialized Women: The Contest in India. *American Ethnologist*, 16(4):622–633.
Das, V. (1986). *The Word and the World: Fantasy, Symbols and Records*. New Delhi, India: Sage Publications.
ICMR (Ministry of Health and Family Welfare). (2005). *National Guidelines for Accreditation, Supervision and Regulation of ART Clinics in India*. Retrieved from http://icmr.nic.in/art/art_clinics.htm on 31st January, 2016.

ICMR (Ministry of Health and Family Welfare). (2010). *The Assisted Reproductive Technologies (Regulation) Bill – 2010*. Retrieved from http://icmr.nic.in/guide/ART%20 REGULATION%20Draft%20Bill1.pdf on 31st January, 2016.

Jejeebhoy, S. (1998). Infertility in India – Levels, patterns and consequences: priorities for social science research. *Journal of Family Welfare*, 44(2):15–24.

Kabeer, N. (2001). Conflicts Over Credit: Re-Evaluating the Empowerment Potential of Loans to Women in Rural Bangladesh. *World Development*, 29(1):63–84.

Khanna, A. (2006). *In other words – sexuality and assisted reproductive technologies: thoughts from a queer perspective*. Monograph commissioned by SAMA. New Delhi, India: SAMA – Resource Group for Women and Health.

Prakasamma, M. (1999). Infertility: A social and gender perspective, *National Consultation on Infertility Prevention and Management*. New Delhi, India: UNFPA.

Reddy, S. & Qadeer, I. (2010). Medical Tourism in India: Progress and Predicament?, *Economic and Political Weekly*, 45(20):69–75.

SAMA. (2010). *Constructing Conception: The Mapping of Assisted Reproductive Technologies in India*. New Delhi, India.

Uberoi, P. (1990). Feminine Identity and National Ethos in Indian Calendar Art. *Economic and Political Weekly*, 25(17):41–48.

Unisa, S. (1999). Childlessness in Andhra Pradesh, India: Treatment seeking and consequences. *Reproductive Health Matters*, 7(13):54–64.

4 A socio-anthropological reflection on infertility and ARTs in Algeria

Aïcha Benabed

Introduction

The social impact of ARTs in Algeria does not appear to be taken seriously into account by either social science specialists or public health authorities. ART, however, has led to the development of certain kinds of social exclusion. It causes considerable difficulties (family, financial, etc.) for many men and women suffering from infertility. ART confronts everyone with the question of their origins, and it also questions the very foundations of Algerian society. In a context of globalisation, the technique is expanding and becoming established as a solution for sterile couples. While the procedure is currently becoming more widespread in the Algerian medical field, it appears to have had little impact on the Algerian family code.

In this chapter we analyse the medical and social application of the procedure in the Algerian context, dominated by the patriarchal and normative ideology governing the status of the mother. Our study seeks to shed light on the norms of access to ART, drawing on the experiences of women who underwent this still uncertain and experimental technique and wanted to escape from the fatality of childlessness.

The introduction of ART led to doubts regarding the patriarchal ideology governing social behaviours, as it questions values based on virility. This ideology supports the need to give birth to a child, since a woman is not considered as such unless she gives birth to a child, or children, after a legally consummated marriage. The child holds a central place in the Algerian family's life. Spouses opt for ART in as much as it is accessible within the legal framework in Algeria, while avoiding conflict with cultural and/or religious values. The social order permits all reproductive techniques provided they are applied to the spouses' own gametes. According to Ossoukine (2007):

> The questions that are put to medical ethics are closely related to life, sex and death, and are also related to the Islamic religion. Two decades previously, North African religious authorities, together with those in the Near and Middle East, decided to meet and to give answers to questions on advances in technology and the sciences and their application to the person. Similarly, religion can be only one of the sources of ethical reflection, or rather a

reference to inspire those reflecting. If ethical questions raised by the development of biotechnologies found answers in the divine texts, bioethics would have no reason for existence. When it intervenes in discussions that involve bioethics, religion may be either in conflict or in convergence with other disciplines.

(Ossoukine, 2007, p. 169)

Moreover, the practice of ART is seen as a complex social fact in the field of medical procreation. It is not a simple technical and biomedical act. Because infertility in some way affects the sense of marital and social relationships, its treatment by means of ART, which is still experimental, takes on social importance. This facet of the issue often plays a part in the distress, stigma and despair of infertile couples.

Our perspective is mainly based on the theory of the sexual and social relationships of infertility and the new reproductive technologies. Engeli (2010, p. 22) stated: "It is as if ART calls into question the vocation of women, with maternity being the traditional heteronormative pattern of the family." The experience of infertility, family pressures and women's demands on medical power act in accordance with social norms that correspond to sexual roles and to powers over the sexes. This means that social and medical institutions exert influence on the patients. ART treatment and its development are part of a relationship of social influence, with social control on procreation. Changes that may occur in the relationship between the sexes can only be perceived through analysing transformations taking place in the institutions that are responsible for ensuring the continuity of the gender order, such as the family, school and religion.

Our reflection is based on a qualitative survey carried out in three medical facilities in the city of Oran[1] and in western Algeria (one in the public sector and two in the private sector). These facilities were selected for study because they are most representative of ART practice in the west of the country. In the public hospital centre, only one artificial insemination technique was used. The women undergoing investigations came from all provinces of Algeria. We carried out repeated one-to-one interviews with a series of 18 couples, two gynaecologists, a lawyer and a biologist. The present paper draws only on the interviews with the women concerned. In the same situation, men were less willing to cooperate on their own and to talk about their childless marital life, about fathering children and sexuality. Men are reticent when speaking of their intimate life. Patients were selected from a variety of social statuses (age, educational level, standard of living and background). Their ages ranged between 24 and 42 years. Some cases involved male factor infertility, where physiological problems were detected, while in others the origin of infertility was not identified and the specialists admitted that they were unable to offer a solution.

In this chapter we also propose, firstly, to describe the overall context of ART, subject to the inescapable social norms that govern procreation. Then, through the experiences of some women consulting for ART, we will show that only the woman constantly undergoes regular consultations and medical examinations, whereas the man rarely attends. Childless women are considered as women who do not fit the gender norms.

ART, an increasingly important social reality

Procreation holds a foremost rank among the statutory values of the Algerian family. Delay in having a child quickly leads to tensions and conflicts in the couple's life and the life of the whole family. Husbands and wives are certainly aware that time is running out for them; society will remind them of this. Not bearing children is a bad experience for the couple and, consequently, it is the woman who is stigmatised by the family circle. The woman is still to blame when deprived of procreation. She suffers twice: because she does not bear children, and because her body is sick. Compelled by social pressures, the couple attempt all available means, in particular ART.

In Algeria, the practice of ART began early in the 1990s, in the public hospital in Algiers, the Hussein Dey University Hospital Centre, by Professor Laliam and Dr Ftouki. Nine live births by in vitro fertilisation were recorded during that period. The practice was then discontinued due to the civil unrest in Algeria in the 1990s. After 2000, ART was reintroduced in some regions of the country. In Oran, little Doha, the first in vitro baby was born on July 14, 2004, by means of artificial insemination in the centre of El Mawloud. Before 2005,[2] only the conscience of the ART Centre team played the role of censor vis à vis all the requests that could be made for such techniques, such as a demand from a menopausal woman, or from a widow who wanted to recover the cryopreserved sperm of her late husband, or couples who wanted their frozen embryos.

Faced with such complex questions, an individual conscience may fail. Following the ordinance n° 05-02 of February 27, 2005, amending and supplementing the law n° 84-11 of June 9, 1984, relating to the family code, the Algerian legislator established ART as a medical technique for procreation controlled by the law for the protection and promotion of health, by the medical ethical code and the religious text. Sperm banks are not available and are prohibited in Algeria, as such a procedure is considered to be adultery. The same prohibition applies to sex selection of the child. Physicians confirmed that some patients with no religious and/or moral objections and who have the means to do so may leave for countries with less strict legislation on ART, such as Jordan, even though it is an Islamic country.

Currently, ART is a social reality which is becoming increasingly present. The process encountered a favourable echo and is rapidly expanding due to the multiplication of centres for reproductive medicine. These now number nine, two of which are in public hospitals (in Algiers and Oran), and seven in private clinics (three in Oran, two in Algiers, one in Annaba and one in Constantine). So the practice is largely reliant on the private sector, which is prepared to meet the growing demand from applicants in Algeria. Before the establishment of the private sector, infertile couples had to go abroad for ART treatment, mainly to Tunisia, at considerable expense.

In Algeria, ART is not destined to increase the size of the population or the index of fecundity. Its avowed aim is to enable infertile couples to have a child in vitro. According to statistics from the Ministry of Health, Population and Hospital Reform, more than 300,000 Algerian couples, or 7% of all couples, suffer from infertility (2002 data). In a number of interviews, gynaecologists have stated that 65% of infertility is due to male factors, compared with a universal mean of 40%. Other specialists in the field, however, deny these data and claim that there has been no real census or any serious studies on infertility in the country so far. There are no statistics on children born by IVF. Women who have successfully undergone IVF give birth in public or private medical facilities outside the ART centres. Births following this technique are seldom declared as such. The legitimacy of ART has rarely been publicly contested, but this has not always been the case. Recourse to such practices has long been kept secret by the couples involved and also by physicians.

Norms and conditions for access to ART

Physicians only carry out assisted procreation in a marital context, as advocated by the Islamic religion. Recourse to ART is authorised only if some conditions are met. These techniques are new to Muslim society, and so former Islamic jurists could not anticipate and provide us with a text or texts ruling the practice. Preserving the lineage (*sulala*) is a part of the essential questions in Islam: honour, religion, the person, property. The child must imperatively be biologically affiliated to the father, for paternity is a sacred matter. Bearing this in mind, it is important to lay down criteria with regard to ARTs. First, the applicant couple must be married legally and according to the precepts of Islam. Second, the ovule of the woman must be fertilised only with the sperm of the husband. Islamic ethics do not allow recourse to the process with cells other than those of one and the same couple. So concerning sperm, a donor other than the husband, whether anonymous or known, is strictly prohibited by Islam. It is impossible to resort to the donation of sperm, ovules or embryos. Islam emphasises the preservation of affiliation (*ennassab*). It is in this spirit that *chariàa* (Islamic law) laid down that the widow or divorced woman should abstain from any sexual relation for three months and ten days before she could marry again, the purpose being to prevent any ambiguity as to affiliation. In Algeria and in Morocco, polygamy is authorised under some conditions. Surrogacy is prohibited. It is permitted in other Muslim countries on condition that the surrogate is the husband's second wife and that he has given his sperm to fertilise the ovule of the first wife. In Tunisia, such a procedure is not possible because polygamy is prohibited (Zerradi, 2009).

As explained above, the relationship must be within a legal marriage. We witnessed a situation where a couple wedded by the *Fatiha*[3] (a statement pronounced by an imam to declare a couple married) was refused when they wished to have ART treatment. Both partners must be present when gametes are fertilised or embryos implanted, acts for which written consent is duly co-signed by the partners before they are performed.

Physicians first emphasise that the centres making decisions with regard to ART must apply the legal texts in relation to this activity, and that ART centres should be created in every town in the country, particularly in areas which have a high rate of infertility. They explain that, ideally, in each Maghreb country a national agency of bioethics should be created to collect data on ART and on organ transplants. This agency should include medical practitioners, biologists, paediatricians, Islamic scholars and jurists.

ART professionals, lawyers and Islamic scholars (*oulemas*[4]) took part in a number of conferences held by the Algerian High Islamic Council in Algiers in order to discuss the issue of Islamic ethics and ARTs. They called for the adoption by each Maghreb country of a national ART register, which would oblige each centre to keep an open register recording its results, and which could be verified by the appropriate authorities. An identical register should be used in all Maghreb countries. The question of the religious norm is frequently cited by the couples, indicating that moral values are deeply rooted in the conscience and mentality. Marriage is deemed to be the "only legitimate source of the formation of the family institution". According to the couples interviewed and who were considering ART as a possible solution, only the sperm of the spouse may be used.

> My wife suggested we should go abroad, yes, I can afford it, it is not a question of money, but I refuse, I refuse because I am not sure of the fertilising agents used, and I'm not sure if the sperm would be mine ... I refuse to call into question the foundations of my family unit ... We have to accept the fact of living without children rather than go forward into uncertainty and disrupt the balance of the family and society...
>
> Company director, 45

Only biological affiliation is accepted for the practice to be performed. Couples consider that insemination by a donor rather than by the legitimate husband can cause confusion within the family. It can also break the natural bonds between parents and offspring, and would ineluctably make affiliation a random matter (Beddiar, 1993). It would have a negative influence on parental status and create conflict with sociocultural norms and values. The maxim often repeated by most couples is that "sperm is a sacred thing; it cannot be donated to a third person". Any pregnancy conceived outside the legal couple is equivalent to adultery and inevitably leads to divorce.

ART practised exclusively in the private sector

ART remains an exclusive practice for the private sector. The private sector replaces the public sectors in all areas in a society newly open to the market economy. The advent of foreign specialists and the importation of advanced technological equipment and expensive drugs creates a market in infertility. This lucrative domain interests both the pharmaceutical industry and laboratories. However, ART is still not taught at the Algerian Faculty of Medicine. Physicians rely on their own resources to find training and refresher courses abroad, so that on their return they can implement this technique. In our interviews with experts, they often suggested introducing ART in the gynaecology teaching programme, so that the procedure will become known in the appropriate departments. While today ART specialists have mastered the techniques of in vitro fertilisation, microinjection and vitrification, couples on the other hand have enormous difficulties in financing their care.

The imported technology used by ART centres requires considerable financial outlay. Costly drugs manufactured by Anglo-Saxon laboratories are required. Likewise, artificial insemination, where injections in vitro remain expensive and are not reimbursed by the social insurance system, is still not treated as a medical act. Physicians constantly ask for these acts to be reimbursed. Only drugs used to stimulate ovulation are reimbursed to women by the social insurance system. As the director of a fertility centre stated:

> The cost ... for example, even if we look only at the practical side of the laboratory, the analyses, even the work involved ... that comes to about 900 to 1,000 euros ... the treatment is reimbursed for people who have insurance of course; for those who don't have insurance, well, it's true that it's rather hard on the purse; you need to know that treatment costs more than 1,000 or 1,500 euros, but it is also true that we have patients from all social backgrounds, you know that for a child, people are ready to spend all that they have.

A physician from another well-known centre said:

> The price of the treatments prescribed can vary by 100%. The same molecule with the same effectiveness may be sold at two different prices. One laboratory supplies it at 37 euros and another at 70 euros. One cycle of treatment can then cost 100 euros to 400 euros, while another costs 800 euros.

It is important to emphasise the distress of infertile couples. They suffer from an injustice in the reimbursement of medical expenses. Expenses are fully reimbursed to those covered by the social security of the armed forces. Reimbursements for other patients apply only to some treatments. Couples with an average income hope that medical acts will be reimbursed for a total of three attempts, as they are for members of the armed forces.

Non-reimbursement of medical acts is a problem and is an obstacle to the spread of ART, and also it does not encourage couples to repeat the attempt in the event of failure. Physicians as well as couples emphasise the need to include ART on the list of treatments that are reimbursed, for three attempts at least. The treatments prescribed are too expensive and are only available to women under the age of 43 years. In vitro fertilisation does not have its rightful place among the techniques and treatments covered by social insurance. This situation places physicians in a true dilemma.

The law does not oblige us to carry out six inseminations before going on to IVF, we don't do that. Even the new WHO standards, which talk of 4%, are not applied in France. So we don't agree with such standards, and we work with the standards of our centre. In fact, these are still recognised, it is David's first classification, well, we made a few changes regarding motility and vitality, but concerning normal sperm we haven't changed but stayed with 3%, one can take an overall value of 20% normality but we never go below 20%; the 4% level laid down by WHO can't be applied in our population.

A biologist

Some couples have recourse to ART discreetly, because if it were known, it would lead to marital conflict. Behind this discretion lies the coercive ideology of the family-in-law, the mother-in-law in particular, who sees these procreation techniques as incompatible with traditional norms and human nature, and so the wider family and society will suspect the affiliation of the child born through this technique. In the opinions of some, a child conceived by ART is a "child created by science", a "chemical child" or a "syringe child". Infertility means social stigmatisation for couples, and primarily for women. ART helps couples to achieve their project of having a natural child, reflecting their perception of the child's role in their life (Bassand and Kellerhals, 1975, p. 10).

ART, a matter for women

When a couple is unable to procreate, it is always the woman who undergoes the majority of investigations and treatments. Women try by all available means to overcome their infertility. They sometimes have to go through long and painful courses of treatment, the outcome of which is uncertain. It is often during the workup of the couple's infertility that the male factor is identified. Recourse to ART is burdensome. After a few months of marriage, women undergo strong pressure from their respective families to produce a child, from their mothers-in-law in particular. They believe that all marriages must produce children. This notion was expressed in our interviews. As Naima explained:

When you marry, you marry your family-in-law ... In Algeria, we are not only a husband and a wife, we are married to the family, the family-in-law, because infertility is not only a question of the couple, but a family problem, and one of lineage.

Children evidently play a central role in family life. Sakina, who already has a little girl and wants to give birth to a child by IVF, confesses:

I would like to have a second child, because having only one child is not well considered. People always remind you that the child needs a little brother or sister, and even I don't like to see my daughter alone; she needs a brother to protect her.

The major role of a woman is to ensure the family lineage. She must assume maternity and her duty towards society. Works such as those of Francoise Héritier (1996) highlighted that it is through marriage that men become fathers. In most societies, "the rule is that the husband of the mother is the father of the children". In this context, maternity is the only means for women to be recognised by society, and the absence of children can break the marital bond (Héritier, 1996, p. 332).

From a social point of view, the life experiences and challenges which surround infertility are largely dependent on values and interpretations which revolve around the child and the position that the child holds within the family. In the course of a couple's life, infertility is experienced as a disrupting factor which jeopardises the stability and quality of the social relationships of those concerned (Greil, 2002). It is also a state which makes it impossible for the couple to achieve their fundamental desire, "to have a child, to become parents, and so to take their place in the chain of the generations" (Perret, 1994, p. 131).

Infertility and courses of ART treatment

When sterile couples have exhausted all the traditional treatment approaches, they turn to medically assisted procreation. This is a last resort and a costly one, offering only a small chance of success at the price of physical, psychological and financial sacrifices. Couples feel lost in the medical labyrinth; they continually waste time waiting for results and they spend money on fruitless consultations, investigations that are often not properly done, and treatments that are not effective. All this does not encourage them to continue treatment, and even recourse to ART may often lead to failure; the results are disappointing. Couples who are in fact sub-fertile are also labelled as sterile, when in fact they could be treated. They become candidates for IVF. These couples believe that they were not properly cared for, and in particular that they had not found "good" specialists, or sometimes that they had come across "incompetent" ones, who had referred them to private clinics for artificial insemination or to ART centres.

ARTs place the patients and their gynaecologists in an increasing spiral of treatments and a more and more pressing demand for a child. Women are more implicated in the medicalisation of procreation because they are directly involved in the medical interventions, even if the man proves infertile. In spite of the inconveniences of the treatments which affect their body and their personal or professional life, these women accept the constraints of undergoing ART. Infertility cannot be reduced to a simple medical and biological state, because women do not speak of their procreative difficulties in a technical way, but they approach them in relation to identity and to family and affiliation. Infertility reflects a question of social status. So, the value given to the child intervenes in the way infertility is experienced and influences how couples see the new assisted reproductive technologies.

Courses of ART treatment involve only the women and their body, leaving men in the background. Very few husbands choose to be near their wives and they are rarely present. Marked gender imbalance is observed in medical care. Men are rarely involved; they attend only for sperm collection at the ART centre and to sign the consent form, a legal document agreeing to the transfer. Women told us that sometimes physicians arrange the formalities so that the husband does not need to be present.

Most women or couples who seek treatment for infertility have taken this step in a climate of emergency. Couples have difficulty in imagining their life without a child, especially when social pressure is strong. Their relations embarrass them by enquiring whether a baby is on the way. Couples find that some gynaecologists increase their feelings of guilt instead of relieving their distress. As stated by the head of the obstetrics and gynaecology department of Oran public hospital (EHU Oran):

> The doctors I visited all told me the same tale: after the age of 35 you should not wait too long for things to happen naturally. Time is against you after the age of 40. When you reach the menopause, the situation becomes desperate; there is no miracle cure ... Men are increasingly infertile, because their sperm becomes defective and insufficient. Their spermatozoids are damaged by alcohol and cigarettes in particular, but also by other factors such as pollution ... They are soldiers, policemen, gendarmes or drivers. There is certainly a link between profession and infertility ... To me, infertility is becoming an occupational disease.

Physicians observe that in most couples who consult, the woman has been affected by an infection which is common in Algeria, although there have been no reliable studies. Fallopian tube inflammation, of infectious origin, particularly affects young women under 25 years of age. In other words, single women are concerned because they pay less attention to fecundability. They are unaware of the infection and so in the majority of cases it is not treated. Where men are concerned, according to gynaecologists, certain occupations are at higher risk of reduced sperm motility, e.g. bakers, welders. Professional stress also has its share of responsibility in male infertility, while tobacco and alcohol play a considerable part. After each cycle, these women and men who wish to have a child find themselves confronted with failure.

Professionals consider ART as a means of relieving the distress of most infertile couples, to the detriment of preventive efforts that could eliminate some causes of infertility. The constraints involved are not their concern. Some professionals see that patients who come for consultation have chosen ART as the last chance of achieving their parental project. A biologist and head of an ART centre told us:

> In the patients' minds, the ART centre is the last resort, and if it does not work this would be a catastrophe, that is the way they think ... so right from the first consultation, these patients get worried. It is the end, they know very well that this is the last chance, and so they have great difficulty in coping with their stimulation treatment ... and whatever these women are, even if they are doctors, it is difficult for them. The pressure is so strong, whatever

the social status, the family unit is not complete if she doesn't have children, even if the woman is a minister and she doesn't have a child, it's as though she wasn't married, she doesn't have the status of a married woman…

Women who resort to ART describe the procedure as being costly and painful, with the fear of not obtaining a positive result and of possibly having other disorders, the strain of undergoing constant tests and finding excuses for absence from work and also of finding the money to achieve their goal. It is women's bodies that have to be treated even if the infertility comes from the man. Women undergoing a course of ART need to devote enormous time and energy to doctors' visits, examinations, injections and more health risks such as repeated miscarriages.

Women do not feel that doctors listen to them enough. We found no psychologists in ART centres. Women, therefore, do not have the opportunity to talk, which would give them moral and/or social support. The waiting room is, however, a space where women have the opportunity to express their feelings. It is a space where they can share experiences, to alleviate the stigmatisation that affects childless couples. Even when the physician is an attentive listener, working conditions make it impossible to deal with the patient's psychological distress, because he or she cannot concentrate on what the patient is trying to express but only on the physical symptoms.

Physicians do not take into account the occupational constraints of professional women. They only take their patients' working conditions into account in so far as these conditions may affect infertility. The appointments planned by the ART centre may not fit in with work timetables. Women state that the need to reconcile their infertility treatment and their professional obligations creates considerable stress. Women must show their commitment, their availability and reliability at work. Souad, a school teacher, underwent two artificial inseminations and an IVF attempt. Repeated absences for consultations and unforeseeable hospitalisations put her in a difficult situation and forced her to conceal her use of ART (just as other patients do).

Women keep silent about ART treatments to protect their careers. Amel, a young woman aged 35, is an engineer at the oil company Sonatrach; she told us:

> My colleague and I have exactly the same diplomas but I have been working for longer than him. When I asked for promotion in my career, the committee's response was favourable, but in front of the boss, my colleague opposed me by telling me that I have been absent too much recently … whereas he knew that I went away for ART treatment.

Women are afraid that they will be dismissed if they reveal to their employer that they have used ART. ART can lead to failure as it places women outside the procreative standard (Rozée and Mazuy, 2012, p. 7). The failure of the technique is perceived as a failure of performance, of the performance of the reproductive bodies (which do not "obey" any longer), but especially as a testing of gender roles (Butler, 2005).

For some women, failure of ART can be very damaging and can have serious side-effects on the couples subjected to this stressful experience. Very often, the couple cannot bear any more disappointment, and a breakup ensues. On the other hand, if infertility is due to the husband, few couples in this situation opt for adoption.[5] Other couples place their hope in a series of repeated attempts to have a child, to avoid feelings of guilt. Women say that as long as ART practice exists and that they have the opportunity to use it, they do so in order to avoid regrets in the future; thereafter, they can wait until a natural pregnancy occurs. Young women believe that after several IVF attempts, their bodies are stimulated and they nurture the hope that a pregnancy will, one day, occur naturally and joy will come to their homes thanks to IVF treatment.

Conclusion

ART involves multiple actors, among them physicians (or gynaecologists), biologists and the couples themselves, in particular the women, in a momentous space of norms relating to procreation and the child. The context in which new reproductive technologies are practised can only be fully grasped through reflection on what childbearing means in our society and how children should be borne. ART is practised against a background of religious norms and gender norms. Failed attempts set the infertile couple outside procreative norms and the norms of Algerian society. Gender norms and sociocultural moral values are inalienable in Algerian society. However, infertility is always thought of as a female matter. ART brings into play a broad spectrum of interventions on the woman's body. However, even if male infertility is involved, it is always the women who come for a diagnosis. Men rarely agree to submit to medical investigations. It is always the woman's body which is subject to intervention.

Notes

1 Oran is a coastal city in western Algeria, the second largest city after the capital. It has three private clinics offering ART (El Mawloud, Makhsane Asrar and Anis) and one ART department in a public hospital, providing care for infertile couples from the immediate area as well as other areas and countries (Maghrebis, Africans and migrants). Various techniques are used: IC, IVF, ICSI. The private centres are equipped for the freezing of sperm and embryos.
2 Art. 11. The law n° 84-11 of June 9, 1984 is supplemented by article 45 (a) as follows: "Art. 45 (a): The two spouses can resort to artificial insemination. Artificial insemination is subject to the following conditions: The marriage must be legal. Insemination must be done with the consent of both spouses. The spermatozoa of the husband and the ovule of the wife must be used, and not those of any other person. Artificial insemination may not take place through a surrogate mother."
3 A *Fatiha* marriage is a religious ceremony. It is not under the control of a civil body.
4 *Oulémas* are religious scholars.
5 In Algeria, adoption is represented by *kafala*, ruled by the executive decree n° 92-24 of January 13th, 1992, modifying the decree n° 71-157 of June 3rd, 1971, relating to name change.

References

Bassand, M., Kellerhals, J. (1975). *Familles urbaines et fécondité.* Geneva: Georg.

Beddiar, A. (1993). *Le regard de l'Islam sur les procréations médicalement assistées.* Paris: AELF Editions.

Butler, J. (2005). *Trouble dans le genre. Pour un féminisme de la subversion.* Paris: La Découverte [1st English ed.: *Gender Trouble: Feminism and the Subversion of Identity.* New York: Routledge, 1990].

Engeli, I. (2010). *Les politiques de la reproduction. Les politiques d'avortement et de procréation médicalement assistée en France et en Suisse.* Paris: L'Harmattan.

Greil, A.L. (2002). Infertile Bodies: Medicalization, Metaphor, and Agency, in *Infertility Around the Globe: New Thinking on Childlessness, Gender, and Reproductive Technologies,* M.C. Inhorn and F.V. Balen (eds). Berkeley: University of California Press, pp. 101–118.

Héritier, F. (1996). *Masculin / Féminin. La pensée de la différence.* Paris: Odile Jacob.

MSPRH, ONS, LEA. (2004). Enquête algérienne sur la santé de la famille 2002. Alger: Ministère de la santé et de la réforme hospitalière, Office national de la statistique et Ligue des États arabes (The Pan Arab Project for Family Health).

Ossoukine, A. (2007). Le comité d'éthique algérien face à la concurrence bureaucratique et religieuse. *Journal International de Bioéthique,* 18(1–2):167–176.

Perret, Z. (1994). Stérilité masculine et transmission de la filiation en procréation médicalement assistée avec donneur. *Ethnologie Française,* 24(1):130–134.

Rozée, V., Mazuy, M. (2012). L'infertilité dans les couples hétérosexuels: genre et "gestion" de l'échec. *Sciences Sociales et Santé,* 30(4):5–30.

Zerradi, M. (2009). Les enjeux éthiques potentiels de la procréation médicalement assistée dans les pays musulmans, cas du Maroc. Available online from www.iireb.org/fichiers_rapports/2009_Zerradi_Mouna.pdf

5 Knowledge and awareness of men about infertility and their involvement in fertility treatment[1]

Rural men's voices from Andhra Pradesh, India

Sucharita Pujari & Sayeed Unisa

Introduction

Infertility is said to be a problem of the reproductive system affecting men and women equally (Ali et al. 2011). Inability to have a child is a source of distress for many couples socially as well as psychologically (Malhlstedt 1985; Greil 1997; Unisa 2001; Widge 2004). It is said that infertile couples display significantly higher psychopathology in the form of tension, hostility, anxiety, depression, self-blame and suicidal tendencies (Unisa 2001; Khan 2001) as compared to couples with children. Studies in Latin American and African countries show that there is a strong social stigma attached to infertility, and often infertile couples are excluded from many social activities and traditional ceremonies (Ali et al. 2011).

Studies in the Indian context also show that a male partner in a marital relationship is often emotionally disturbed if he has been diagnosed to have defects leading to infertility of the couple. Most often men hesitate to visit a health provider for fear of being ridiculed (Mehta and Kapadia 2008). In patriarchal societies even contemplating the idea of infertility in men is rare. Not only is there social pressure on men to prove their virility, but many times, on account of social pressure, childless men have reported having married a second time, while many of them stay away from their wives (Singh, Dhaliwal and Kaur 1996; Unisa 1999; Mehta and Kapadia 2008).

In developing countries, the incidence of preventable infertility is very high compared to developed countries, and in the majority of cases, the causes are identifiable and can be treated (Ali et al. 2011). Based on available literature, in nearly 45% of the cases where the couples are unable to have a child there is male factor infertility (Garner 1997; Inhorn 2003; Mahmood et al. 2005) and the contributing factors generally include poor sperm production due to testicular damage from infection caused by mumps, genetic problems, blockages to sperm ducts due to sexually transmitted infections or congenital defects, consumption of certain drugs, smoking, alcohol, regular heavy drinking, obesity, poor diet and certain occupational exposures to heavy metals or pesticides (Bashed et al. 2012).

Knowledge about infertility is quite poor among men and women in many parts of the world. Couples often have little knowledge about the fertile period and when to seek treatment (Dyer et al. 2004). In addition to the low level of knowledge, there are a number of misconceptions regarding infertility across the globe. In many African countries, for instance, evil forces, eating sweet foods or engaging in sexual intercourse with older women are thought to be responsible for infertility (Okonofua et al. 1997).

It is equally important to emphasize that to be able to integrate both partners in the treatment of infertility, men should have correct knowledge and awareness about the various medical causes of childlessness and the various treatment options.

Gaps in male health literacy in terms of awareness about reproductive issues and infertility can lead to unnecessary anxiety and delays in seeking help and treatment which may lead to worse health outcomes. There is a general notion among men that infertility is primarily a female problem, and many are unaware of the factors which may have already affected their fertility, for instance, being overweight. Though not all causes of infertility can be prevented yet, it is important that males should know that certain infections, mumps for instance, can cause testicular swelling and reduced sperm count, and this is a disease which can be prevented by vaccination. That is also why it is important to keep oneself safe from sexually transmitted infections. Further knowledge of fertility issues can also reduce unnecessary delays in seeking medical help when pregnancy does not occur.

Keeping the above perspective in mind, the present chapter focuses on how men understand infertility and their involvement in seeking fertility treatment, based on a study of married childless males in rural Andhra Pradesh. Not many studies on men's knowledge of and attitudes toward infertility have been conducted in India. Most often the data concerning fertility and childlessness have typically focused on women's experiences, without emphasizing men's role in the infertility management and treatment process.

Materials and methods

Site and study design

To understand the male perspective on infertility, a descriptive community-based study was conducted. Andhra Pradesh was selected firstly because the rate of childlessness was reportedly high there, according to National Family Health Survey figures 1998–99 (NFHS 1998). Secondly, it was easy to identify childless couples in this area as a study on childlessness had already been conducted in the state (Unisa 2001).

The selection of the sample for the present study was drawn from the list of childless couples already identified in a study entitled *Social Psychological Consequences of Childlessness in Andhra Pradesh* carried out during 1996–2001 by the International Institute for Population Studies (IIPS), under the Ford Foundation Grant (Unisa 2001). A descriptive community-based study was conducted with a selected sample of childless men from 30 villages in the Ranga Reddy District of Andhra Pradesh. For this study, the list of the childless couples from the previous survey was modified by including a complete house listing of selected villages and inviting new childless couples for interview. Husbands of women aged 20 years and above, with at least three years of marital duration and childless at the time of data collection, were selected for interview.

A total of 181 interviews were conducted, using a semi-structured pre-tested interview schedule having both closed- and open-ended questions. The data was collected through face-to-face interviews with childless men. The interviews were mostly conducted at interviewees' homes, or at places convenient to the respondents in the native language, by a team of investigators who had undergone intensive training for data collection. Informed consent was taken from all the respondents, and the respondents had the freedom to withdraw at any stage.

Questionnaire

The interview schedule was designed based on previously published literature on men and infertility. The interview schedule was originally designed in English and later translated into Telugu by a professional translator. It was thoroughly discussed with the study team and pre-tested in an urban slum in the city of Hyderabad. Modifications and revisions, wherever required, were then incorporated into the final interview schedule. The interview schedule covered several domains, such as knowledge of reproductive organs, causes of infertility, treatment-seeking pattern attitudes towards ARTs and child adoption (Pujari 2008).

Analysis was carried out in SPSS, and this chapter is based on the results of bivariate, ANOVA and multivariate analyses of dependent variable knowledge and treatment of infertility by socio-economic characteristics of males. ANOVA has been used to explore significant differentials between the variables.

Findings

Socio-demographic characteristics of the sample

The majority of the respondents (55.2%) were aged 30 and above (see Table 5.1). Their mean age at the time of the interview was 36.6 years. Most of them were married for ten years or more, and 77% of them were living in nuclear families. Twelve per cent of these men were in bigamous marriage (their second marriage was primarily due to the inability of getting a child from the first wife); close to one fourth (24.3%) were in consanguineous marriages. Nearly one fifth (20.9%) of the respondents were living with an adopted child.

The majority (90.6%) of the respondents were Hindus; Muslims and Christians constituted 7% and 2% respectively.

One third of the respondents were illiterate (32.5%). Of those who were literate, a large proportion (28.7%) had attained secondary level education. Farming and

Table 5.1 Demographic and socio-economic background of the respondents

Background variables	Percentage	Number of men
Current age		
< 30	35.4	64
30–39	32.0	58
40–49	18.2	33
50+	14.4	26
Mean age	**36.6**	—
Duration of marriage in years		
3 years	12.7	23
4–9 years	37.0	67
10 years and above	50.2	91
Type of family		
Nuclear	77.3	140
Joint	22.7	41
Religion		
Hindu	90.6	164
Muslim	7.2	13
Christian	2.2	4
Caste		
Scheduled caste	32.6	59
Scheduled tribe	3.3	6
OBC	46.4	84
General/Others	17.7	32
Occupation of the respondent		
Agricultural labourer/ Cultivation	48.1	87
Non-agricultural	51.9	94
Education		
Illiterate	32.5	59
Primary	23.2	42
Middle	15.4	28
Secondary and above	28.7	52
Adopted child		
Yes	20.9	38
No	79.0	143
Total	100.0	181

cultivation were the two primary occupations of the men interviewed. Many of them were working as agricultural labourers on others' land. Though non-agricultural workers formed a large part of the sample (52%), they were mostly engaged in low-skilled or unskilled jobs and worked as electricians, mechanics, laundry men, goldsmiths, barbers, stone crushers, etc. About 44% of the respondents' wives were housewives, and only 5% of the respondents reported that their wives were working in the service sector. Most of them belonged to modest households (medium standard of living).

Knowledge about reproductive physiology and fertile period

Research shows that knowledge of infertility is quite inadequate in many parts of the world (Ali et. al. 2011), even among childless couples. Couples are generally unaware of the period of the month in which they are most fertile and when to seek treatment. To assess the knowledge about the correct timing of the fertile period, the respondents in the present study were first asked to name the male and female reproductive organs that they thought played an important role in human reproduction, followed by questions on the length of the menstrual cycle, the timing of the fertile period and the place where the human foetus grows. The results show that 57% men reported correctly about male reproductive organs (penis, testes or both) and of these, a large number of men (40.9%) have exclusively reported the penis as a vital male organ related to reproduction, followed by 4% of men who mentioned the testes. Twenty-seven per cent of men have reported other physiological components such as sperm, chromosomes, semen, etc., as playing an important role in reproduction.

Knowledge about the female organs of reproduction is relatively better, as more than 80% were aware of them, and of these a majority reported the uterus (30%) and vagina (24%) as the vital female organs related to reproduction. For comparative analysis, by background variables we have combined the responses stated for male and female reproductive organs, to see how many reported having some knowledge of reproductive organs and how many had absolutely no knowledge (see Table 5.2). The findings showed that more than 70% of men stated having some knowledge of human reproductive organs. Analysis by levels of education shows that knowledge and awareness about reproductive physiology is far better among men who are literate (79.5%) in comparison to men who have never been to school (55.9%). Those with literate wives (88.4% of the respondents) are more knowledgeable in comparison to men whose wives are illiterate (61.6%). By logistic regression analysis, it was found that those respondents whose wives are literate are three times more likely to have knowledge of reproductive organs in comparison to men whose wives are illiterate. Those with media exposure (76.3%) are two times more likely to have knowledge of reproductive organs compared to men who are never exposed to mass media (48.3%), and it is also statistically significant at the 10% level. The results by treatment variable show that men who have sought treatment (81.2%) are six times more likely to possess knowledge than men who have not sought any treatment (41.9%).

Most of the respondents heard or learnt about reproductive organs either from wives or friends. One third reported that doctors have been their major source of information regarding reproductive organs. Close to 30% could not state any organ associated with human fertility.

It is presumed that the more knowledge a man has, and the better informed he is about human reproductive anatomy and the process of reproduction, the better the

Table 5.2 Percentage of men with knowledge about reproductive organs

Background variables	Knowledge of reproductive organs†	Results of logistic regression		Number of men
		Sig.	B	
Education				
Illiterate ‡	55.9			59
Literate	79.5	.380	1.468	122
Education of the wife				
Illiterate ‡	61.6			112
Literate	88.4	.048	**2.892****	69
Exposure to mass media				
No‡	48.3			29
Yes	76.3	.190	2.089	152
Whether treatment sought				
No ‡	41.9			43
Yes	81.2	.000	**6.202*****	138

† Multiple response answer ; * 10% significant; ** 5% significant; *** 1% significant
‡ Reference category

likelihood of his correctly understanding the nature of the problem of infertility that he or his wife is suffering from, and thereby dealing with it effectively.

The next question concerned knowledge about the fertile period. Men were asked when during the menstrual cycle a woman is most likely to conceive (see Table 5.3). It was found that almost all had correct knowledge about the age when a woman gets her menarche and the correct length of the menstrual cycle. However, very few had correct knowledge about the timing of the fertile period (halfway between two periods). The findings show that only 13.8% of the respondents reported correctly about the fertile period, whereas a majority had no knowledge or incorrect knowledge about the period when women were most fertile. Bivariate analysis showed that men who sought allopathic treatment, and belonged to high socio-economic status (SES) households, with relatively higher levels of education and non-agricultural jobs, had better knowledge about the fertile period compared to their counterparts.

The respondents were posed further questions about the location of the growing foetus and the early signs of pregnancy; 65.7% of the men were aware that the foetus grows inside the uterus. Seventy-eight per cent of the respondents said that missed periods and vomiting are the most common early signs of pregnancy. The higher the level of education of the couple and the more exposure they have to mass media, the better their overall knowledge related to pregnancy. Based on logistic regression analysis, it was observed that education and treatment-seeking has a significant impact on the respondent's knowledge about the location of the growing foetus. Respondents who are literate and who had sought treatment from allopathic doctors are two times more likely to have correct knowledge in comparison to their counterparts.

Table 5.3 Percentage of men with correct knowledge about where the foetus grows by selected background variables

Socio-economic variables	Knowledge about where the baby grows (%)	Results of logistic regression		Number of men
Education		Sig.	B	
Illiterate ‡	47.5			59
Literate	74.6	.046	*2.303***	122
Education of wife				
Illiterate ‡	61.6			112
Literate	72.5	.377	.657	69
SLI				
Low ‡	44.3			61
Medium	69.8	.065	2.238	63
High	84.2	.001	*6.169****	57
Exposure to mass media				
Yes	71.1			152
No ‡	37.9	.225	1.920	29
Whether treatment sought				
Yes	71.7			138
No ‡	46.5	.024	*2.611***	43

* 10% significant; ** 5% significant; *** 1% significant
‡ Reference category

Men's involvement in fertility treatment

Decision making

Fertility-treatment behaviour depends on the notions of reproductive physiology, the pattern of distress and blame and the perceived causes of infertility. Other determining factors are the availability and affordability of various healthcare practitioners and services.

In the present study, one third of respondents realised that there was a problem in conceiving within the first two years of marriage. More than 80% of respondents worried about their wife's constant failure to achieve a pregnancy, which led to depression, tension and anxiety. However, most discussed the problem with their wives, and also shared the problem with parents and in-laws. In India, since bearing a child is primarily thought to be a married woman's responsibility and the failure to conceive puts the burden of treatment on the woman entirely, most of the literature on couple infertility shows that generally the married women in the household take the first step towards visiting a health practitioner for infertility treatment. However, contrary to what the literature says, most of the respondents (63%) in the present research study said that they were actively involved in initiating the process of seeking treatment. In a few instances, this involved a joint decision (18%). Parents in the household are taken into confidence before initiating any treatment process.

On the other hand, when the health providers in the villages were questioned, they took a different stand. On being asked whether the man comes alone or the couple come together for the treatment, it was found that generally the woman visits the local health provider initially and is mostly accompanied by her mother-in-law or her own mother. Initially the husband does not accompany his wife. According to one of the providers, 'Men are very adamant and don't show any interest when it comes to diagnosis and tests. Only after repeated attempts to convince them through their wife, the men come forward for the tests.' It was reported that the man visits the health provider, unaccompanied by his wife, just to enquire if he by any chance is at fault for their inability to have a child. Men often have a preconceived notion that they cannot be at fault. Only after their second marriage when they still cannot bear a child, the realisation dawns that they could be at fault. However, it needs to be mentioned that these things did not come to the light while interviewing the respondents.

The involvement of the respondents in the search for a doctor for the initial treatment is comparable with their involvement in the search for the subsequent treatment sought. For the subsequent treatments, the type of treatment sought is heavily influenced by what others say and recommend.

Type of treatment sought

Out of the 181 childless men who were interviewed, 20% were seeking treatment at the time of the data collection, 57% had discontinued taking treatment and 24% reportedly had not consulted anywhere, though a few of them stated their plans to start treatment soon. Out of the 138 men who went for any treatment (see Table 5.4), most of them (79.7%) visited allopathic doctors for the first consultation. Mostly doctors in private health facilities were preferred. There was a negative feeling towards infertility treatment offered in public health facilities. However, if the treatment did not yield any positive results, alternative treatments from herbalists, ayurveda and religious methods were sought. Religious and traditional methods of treatment were the first choice of only a very few (<10%). Though a large proportion of the respondents still preferred allopathic doctors for the second consultation, the proportion of men (34.7%) significantly declined and alternatively there has been a significant increase in the number of men opting for ayurveda, homeopathy and unani (AHU), traditional or religious methods of treatment. Perhaps due to the high cost incurred at private hospitals for infertility treatment, many of them may have dropped out after the initial consultation, or if they went for further treatment, it has mostly been for herbalist or religious methods of treatment.

Nearly 80% of respondents chose allopathic treatment as their first choice. Further analysis shows that after the first treatment, more than half of these men (56%) did not go for any subsequent allopathic treatment. The main reason for stopping after the first allopathic consultation could have been the rising cost incurred and also the number of visits one needs to undertake. Previous studies of women's fertility-treatment behaviour shows that medical treatment of infertility is generally long-term and couples feel rather disappointed because there are no immediate and visible results (Unisa 1999; Unisa 2001).

Table 5.4 Distribution of men with regard to the type of fertility treatment sought and sequence of choices

Type of health providers visited	Sequence in which treatment was sought (number of men)		
	First choice	Second choice	Third choice and above
Allopathic (private and govt.)	110	24	6
AHU*	5	9	4
Traditional†	11	21	10
Religious practice	12	15	4
Total	**138**	**69**	**24**

*Ayurveda, homeopathy and unani; † Herbal and home remedies

In the present study, many men had stopped seeking treatment because doctors informed them about their respective physiological defects and the difficulty in producing a child. Moreover, previous studies on childlessness and women in the same area also had similar findings: if it was the wife's problem, the husband preferred remarrying instead of going for further treatment (Unisa 2001).

It was also found that the respondents frequently changed doctors (mainly allopathic). The respondents opined that they were not happy with the advice offered by the doctor or did not get satisfactory answers regarding the cause of their inability to have a child, and hence there was a frequent shift from one health provider to another. The findings also show that there has been a gradual decrease in the number of persons choosing the allopathic mode of treatment as the number of courses of treatment increased, with a gradual shift to alternative treatment options. There is also a noticeable decrease in the number of visits per course of treatment sought. The mean number of visits ranged from 8.8 visits for the first course of treatment to 7.4 for the fifth course of treatment and above. This could be because most of the couples gave up hope of having a biological child and discontinued the treatment. The long period of treatment makes the experience extremely stressful and confusing for many men, as a result of which there is a constant change of doctors largely due to impatience of the couples.

Knowledge about reproductive physiology and line of treatment chosen

We also assessed whether knowledge about the reproductive system and the fertile period is linked with the type of treatment sought by the respondents. The analysis shows a positive association between knowledge about the reproductive system and the choice of treatment sought. It is observed that more than 80% of men who sought allopathic treatment were well informed about the biological causes of infertility and the fertile period as compared to their counterparts. Thus it clearly shows that the greater the awareness and knowledge about the correct functioning of the reproductive physiology, the greater the inclination towards seeking allopathic treatment.

In addition to the above, economic, occupational and educational status of the respondents also determined the type of treatment sought. Those who belonged to high SES households and who had high levels of education sought treatment from private allopathic doctors. By occupational status, more men engaged in non-agricultural occupations preferred the allopathic mode of treatment compared to other methods of treatment.

Financial burden of treatment leading to discontinuation of treatment

Lack of money for funding the treatment invariably stands as an obstacle for those wanting to seek any method of treatment, allopathic or non-allopathic. The respondents in the present study had visited temples, performed religious rituals and offered prayers by paying some amount of money to the priest in their attempt to have a biological child. Deeper probing revealed that quite a significant amount of money was invested in travelling (especially if the doctor's clinic was far away from the village), in paying the doctor's fees, in buying medicine and in boarding and lodging expenses. Most of the respondents (64%) perceived this as a financial burden, and had stopped seeking treatment as it was getting difficult to purchase the prescribed medicine, to undertake the basic diagnostic tests and to pay the doctors' fees. Many of them said that there was 'no sign of positive results' i.e. there was no sign of pregnancy.

The respondents stated they had to borrow money and sell household property to be able to meet the expenses. Some respondents were in debt and had absolutely no money left for treatment at the time of interview. These men were waiting with hopes that very shortly they would restart the treatment once the arrangements for money were in place.

The analysis of mean cost by type of treatment shows that those who went to government hospitals (public hospitals) on average spent nearly 3,000 rupees; that included the cost of travel and diagnostic tests. On the other hand, the average expenditure on treatment from private clinics and hospitals was as high as 12,500 rupees. The cost increased by almost three and a half times for treatment from private hospitals. Despite this fact, the number of men who reported going to private hospitals was very high. The mean cost of other forms of traditional treatment (ayurveda and herbal) is close to 2,500 rupees. Unisa's (2001) study reported similar findings, wherein childless women visited private doctors more than doctors at public hospitals. Unisa showed that in public hospitals, though there are no fees for consultations, the pathological and diagnostic equipment required for various tests for treating infertility is not available, and that becomes the primary reason for seeking treatment at private hospitals and clinics.

Logistic regression analysis was carried out to understand the effect of socio-demographic variables on seeking treatment, and the findings show that a large number of men in the 30–39 age group have sought treatment, which is statistically significant. Men who have some support, either financial or moral, are four times more likely to seek treatment than men who do not have any support, and it is statistically significant at 1%. Men with correct knowledge of reproductive organs are six times more likely to seek treatment than men without any knowledge of reproductive organs. More than 80% of the respondents sought advice from a health provider because they genuinely wanted to have a child, whereas 16% sought treatment due to pressure from family members, including their wife.

Awareness about ARTs

Knowledge and awareness about ARTs was also assessed. Of the respondents, 33.7% were aware of ARTs. Overall, there is a negative attitude towards ARTs as a treatment option. Men are largely ignorant about ARTs. Those who are aware do not prefer them because of the cost factor and also due to the unavailability of these facilities in public hospitals. So far as attitudes towards ARTs go, the reactions were varied. Many had reservations about the high cost of treatment and preferred the natural mode of conception. On the other hand, there were some who were quite optimistic and were positive about these methods. Except for three men, a majority had never tried these treatment methods. It also needs to be mentioned that for some, money was not a problem; some of them were ready to go to any extent, including borrowing and selling household items, which many of them have done, in order to have their own biological child. However, in such cases, distance and reaching out to the doctor turned out to be a problem. Many times the doctor was not available all the time and posed further problems in terms of time and money. Many wanted to make use of these methods, but could not do so, because of the location of the clinic. The respondents felt that very few could actually afford modern treatment methods, as they were accessible in private hospitals and clinics in the distant cities. Child adoption was viewed negatively. Only 12% had adopted a child and none of them wanted to recommend adopting a child to others.

Discussion and conclusion

Considering the fact that male infertility has been rising in the Indian population in the last couple of years, not just in the urban areas but rural areas as well, it is imperative that the state should consider developing programmes and educative materials that would address the needs of the childless men in the rural areas. Men are often ignorant and lack knowledge about the fact they could be also at fault in their inability to have a child. Though our findings showed that a majority agreed with the view that either the man or woman could be the cause of childlessness, informal discussions and deeper probing revealed that a large number of the respondents held the view that the woman is primarily responsible for childlessness.

It is important that basic knowledge of the human reproductive system should be imparted along with a basic understanding of the fertile period, even to the general population, besides incorporating information on physical and lifestyle factors leading to infertility. It is important that men should be informed on linkages between sexually transmitted infections, excessive smoking and alcohol, and infertility.

Most often in infertility treatment, the women in the family blame themselves for not achieving a pregnancy, and most of the time they visit the doctor accompanied by their mothers-in-law or mothers. Husbands may or may not accompany their wives in their first visit to the doctor. Sensible gender-sensitive awareness campaigns with regard to causes of infertility should be developed. Men have many misconceived ideas and notions of infertility, which do not allow them to accept that they may also be at fault. It is therefore important to educate men that fertility treatment involves participation from both husband and wife. Gender-sensitive counselling should be adopted by the state health functionaries while counselling childless couples.

Lack of information about where to seek advice was the major reason for those who did not seek any treatment. There are no special government interventions to treat infertile couples at present, and thus intervention in terms of educating the community about fertility clinics and hospitals would help childless couples to access effective medical care and deal with their childlessness. Many of them have reported that even if certain basic diagnostic tests are made available in public hospitals, it would mean saving a great deal of money, which could be used later for treatments at referral hospitals. It is equally important to educate and counsel family members and elders in the household about the different treatment-seeking options, as they are the ones who are taken into confidence before seeking any treatment.

The long period of treatment makes the experience extremely stressful and confusing for many men, as a result of which there is a constant change of doctors largely due to impatience. Strategies should be evolved to discourage childless couples from seeking treatment from multiple healthcare providers.

There is a need to address the negative pressure from family and community about a couple's childlessness. It is also important to dispel any belief that women are invariably at fault.

Based on the study's findings, we conclude that there is a need for community education on the physiology of involuntary childlessness and appropriate counselling of men to educate them on the real causes of infertility and to get them involved in the infertility treatment process. Reproductive health programmes and policies should aim towards imparting knowledge about such issues, along with knowledge about contraception. Social media can play an important role. Television would be an effective medium to target the rural population, who not only have a poor knowledge regarding causes and treatments of infertility, but are more likely to seek alternative treatments. Hence in the light of our findings, further research should be done on ways to improve male participation in infertility management.

Note

1 An abridged version of this paper was presented in a workshop entitled "Are New Reproductive Technologies Beneficial for Women" in the Women's World Congress on Gender in a Changing World, held at the University of Hyderabad, India, 17 – 22 August, 2014.

References

Ali S, Sophie R, Imam A, Khan F, Ali SF, Shaikh A, Farid-ul-Hasnain S. (2011) Knowledge, perceptions and myths regarding infertility among selected adult population in Pakistan: a cross-sectional study. *BMC Public Health* 11:760.

Bashed MA, Alam GM, Kabir MA, Al-Amin AQ. (2012) Male infertility in Bangladesh: What serve better – pharmacological help or awareness programme? *International Journal of Pharmacology* 8: 687–694.

Dyer SJ, Abrahams N, Mokoena NE, van der Spuy ZM. (2004) You are a man because you have children: experiences, reproductive health knowledge and treatment-seeking behaviour among men suffering from couple infertility in South Africa. *Human Reproduction* 19(4):960–967.

Garner C. (1997) Infertility. In Wasserheit Tsui and J Hagga (eds), *Reproductive Health in Developing Countries*. Washington: National Academy Press, pp. 611–628.

Greil, AL. (1997) Infertility and psychological distress: A critical review of the literature. *Social Science and Medicine* 45:1,679–1,704.

Inhorn MC. (2003) The worms are weak: Male infertility and patriarchal paradoxes in Egypt. *Men and Masculinities* 5(3):236–256.

Khan ME. (2001) Infertility: Its causes and consequences in Indian scenario. In Chander P. Puri and Paul Van Look (eds), *Sexual and Reproductive Health: Recent Advances and Future Directions, Vol II*. New Delhi: New Age International Private Limited.

Mahmood A, Prabhakara, MG, Babu, M, Bajaj, V, Manjunath, GB, Vasan, SS, Prasannakumar, KM, Kumar, A. (2005) Cytogenetic and molecular analysis of infertile males from Bangalore, India. In *Proceedings 15th Annual Meeting of ISSRF and Symposium on Trends in Molecular and Applied Approaches to Reproduction*, Kolkata, India.

Malhlstedt P. (1985) The psychological components of infertility. *Fertility and Sterility* 43:335–346.

Mehta B, Kapadia S. (2008) Experiences of childlessness in an Indian context: A gender perspective. *Indian Journal of Gender Studies* 15(3):437–460.

National Family Health Survey. (1998–1999) International Institute for Population Sciences, Mumbai, India.

Okonofua FE, Harris D, Obebiyi A, Kaned T, Snow RC. (1997) The social meaning of infertility in South West Nigeria. *Health Transition Review* 7:205–220.

Pujari S. (2008) An Insight into Men's experiences of Involuntary Childlessness – A Study of Rural Childless Men. In: A Pradesh, Unpublished PhD Thesis. Mumbai, India: International Institute for Population Sciences.

Singh A, Dhaliwal LK, Kaur A. (1996) Infertility in a primary health centre of North India: A follow-up study. *Journal of Family Welfare* 42(1):51–57.

Unisa S. (1999) Childlessness in Andhra Pradesh, India: Treatment-seeking and consequences. *Reproductive Health Matters* 7(13):54–64.

Unisa S. (2001) Sequence of fertility treatment among childless couples in Ranga Reddy district Andhra Pradesh India. *Asia-Pacific Population Journal* 16(2):161–176.

Widge A. (2004) Infertility. In: SJ. Jejeebhoy (ed.), *Looking back and looking forward: A profile of sexual and reproductive health in India*. New Delhi: Population Council.

6 Reproductive roaming

The quest for children of African couples in France

Véronique Duchesne

Introduction

Infertility and childlessness in developing countries are a public health issue that is largely ignored (Rutstein and Shah, 2004). Despite the documented prevalence of infertility, local and international governmental and non-governmental organisations have identified "hyperfertility" and birth spacing, rather than infertility and threatened reproduction, as "population problems" in sub-Saharan Africa. We need to remember that sub-Saharan Africa is disproportionately affected by infertility (Ericksen and Brunette, 1996), owing largely to the problem of untreated reproductive tract infections (Inhorn, 2009). Large portions of central Africa have long been characterised by unusually low fertility (Leonard, 2002; Retel-Laurentin, 1974). Based on post-World War II sample surveys and censuses of varying quality, demographers have identified an "infertility belt" or geographical area of low fertility in sub-Saharan Africa (Tichit, 2009). This "area of variable geometry" covers Sahelian West Africa, Central and East Africa down to Tanzania: most of this area belonged to French Equatorial Africa[1] (Cooper, 2013). African countries are pronatalist (abortion is illegal), but there is no regulation of the practice of ART, and most centres are in private clinics. In this chapter, I will present background information on the experience of infertile African couples and then examine their reproductive mobility.

Methods and data

This study is part of a broader research project on "Sterility and assisted reproductive technologies in a globalized world (Douala, Paris, Pretoria)", coordinated by the anthropologist Doris Bonnet and funded by the Agence Nationale de la Recherche (France).[2] The research methodology for this study gave priority to ethnographic fieldwork (March 2011 to May 2013), using participant observation in a semi-private hospital (east of Paris) and in a physician's office (east of the Île de France region), and interviews in and out of medical settings.[3] In both places I primarily chose to observe gynaecological consultations and ultrasound examinations. In the hospital, I also participated, as an observer, in the first appointment for ART registration, at which both partners were present. Other observations during laboratory consultations, blood sampling, egg retrieval and embryo transfer gave me a global approach to ART use from the patients' viewpoint.

Repeated semi-structured interviews were carried out with five gynaecologists at their workplace. I also conducted 30 ethnographic interviews with their patients who were born in Africa and who agreed to be interviewed about their use of ART: 21 women and seven (heterosexual) couples. Most of the interviews, which lasted between 45 minutes to two and a half hours, were carried out with the woman alone (sometimes with a sister or a young child), less often with both partners. Most interviews took place in a medical setting, while others took place in the couples' homes in the Paris region. Interviews were conducted in French and were recorded. Except for one Ghanaian couple, the interviewees were born in a French-speaking African country: 17 in West Africa (one in Benin, four in Ivory Coast, four in Guinea, five in Mali, two in Senegal, two in Togo); eight in Central Africa (five in Cameroon, three in the Republic of Congo) and three in the Indian Ocean (two in Comoros, one in Mayotte). Four women were in France for transnational reproductive travel and their husbands were at home in Africa (Cameroon, Guinea, Niger and Comoros). I also carried out one interview and several informal exchanges with the husband of one of the women during his short visits to France, and an interview with a woman, born in Benin and living and working in France, who travelled to a clinic in Ghana to become pregnant.

My research data covered persons from various social backgrounds and very different educational levels. Three women had a high school diploma in their home country (Cameroon and Senegal), while one woman from Mali had never been to school and spoke French only with great difficulty. All were working during the study, except the four women who came with a tourist visa. They left their jobs or took leave because of the couple's project to conceive a child through ART. In their home country their occupations were bank employee, trader, official and manager. While women and couples visiting from abroad have to pay for ART, those with a valid residence permit do not. In France, up to three IVF attempts are covered by the social insurance system. With two exceptions, all the women were married or about to get married (religious, civil or customary marriage).

Infertility life courses

Reproduction is a crucial part of the life path for African men and women alike. Fertility and the ability to conceive are core social dimensions. They involve kinship making and also concern political power, especially in rural areas of Africa (Duchesne, 1998; Feldman-Savelsberg, 2002). Even in urban zones, reproduction is an essential feature of marriage. A married couple without a child is stigmatised and is considered "abnormal" (Hörbst, 2012b). The biomedical definition of infertility has limited applicability: any failure to have children or to have them survive until childhood is seen as infertility, as is the failure to fulfil a reproductive ambition, including having children of only one sex or not becoming pregnant more than once or twice (Sundby, 2002). To give birth to a (live) child is an empowerment for women, both among their family-in-law and socially. And "not giving a child" to their husband carries the risk of divorce, or polygymous unions.

In sub-Saharan Africa, huge differences have been observed between women and men in the experiences and implications of infertility and childlessness (Schuster and Hörbst, 2006). In contemporary African societies, the awareness of male infertility seems to have increased (Dyer et al., 2004). While women still bear the major brunt of infertility, men too suffer from stigmatisation and loss of social status due to infertility (Boerma and Mgalla, 2001). Male infertility is generally conflated with sexual impotency and lack of virility (Hörbst, 2008). Infertility is an indicator of women's vulnerability to witchcraft, to occult power used to harm (Feldman-Savelsberg, 2002). The couples interviewed in France did not suggest that their infertility was due to witchcraft, but childless women are stigmatised. Mariama and Moktar had their religious marriage in Senegal in November 2004 and their civil marriage in June 2005 in France. When I interviewed them in their home, Mariama expressed her pain to me in front of her husband: "At family ceremonies or gatherings, every woman comes with her offspring; when you have no child, the way you are looked at is so difficult to bear." Especially since her husband's infertility was diagnosed by the last gynaecologist, she felt this stigmatisation to be an injustice.

Couples living in France are under pressure after marriage, usually by their ascendants, even when the latter are living in Africa (Duchesne, 2014). Mr Sela, 41 years old, came to Europe in 2001, and he has a daughter in his country, Ivory Coast. In France he met his new wife, who also had one daughter in Ivory Coast. They had a customary marriage in 2009 in France, after living together for one year. He talked of his distress when his sister asks over the phone: "When will your wife give birth? We are waiting for your own child." His mother also phones and asks about her grandchildren. He seems despondent because he cannot tell them about the couple's difficulties (in fact his own infertility).

Generally, the couples and the women interviewed do not confide in their ascendants about their difficulties in conceiving, for various reasons; their ascendants have no medical culture and/or they would be morally too affected by their child's infertility. For some women, the family-in-law also pressures them and the quest for a child becomes very important "to save their marriage". Mrs Anta arrived in France after her marriage (customary, religious and civil) in 2004 in Mali. In 2005, with her husband, she had only one daughter, who is in Bamako. She told me that the only chance to "save her marriage" was to have another child: "It seems that my life depends on the birth of a new child." She told me: "I think to myself that soon I will be alone." She added that her father was beginning to ask whether the matrimonial compensation ("bride price")[4] had been paid because if she divorces, he will have to repay it. Her marriage with her "cousin" (the term being a French traduction) is a "preferential marriage" (a class of favourite spouses but not obligated spouses). Filiation is patrilineal and the function of marriage is to assure the continuity of the paternal lineage; in such a case, to conceive a daughter is a sort of infertility, socially speaking. In that case the marriage could end in divorce if no other children are produced. The same expression is observed in the Middle East: "Some Sunni Muslim patients from Lebanon and from other Middle Eastern Muslim countries such as Egypt and Syria are quietly slipping across transnational borders 'to save their marriages' through the use of donor gametes" (Inhorn, 2011: 97).

In France, as in Cameroon, adoption, whether national or international, is not considered a possible alternative by the infertile couple (Bonnet, 2014). Fosterage, the practice of sending children away to be raised by relatives or non-relatives, is very common in Africa and it also exists in a migration context (Kamba and Tillard, 2013). Even when they still have a child in fosterage in their country before coming to France or even in France, couples said that they "need" their "own" child: a child would strengthen their relationship (Hörbst, 2006). For the couples interviewed, what is important is to "produce" their child together, but they made no reference to genetic affiliation.

The same idea, of conceiving their own child, is also expressed by the parents of the couples. François, a Togolese who grew up in Ivory Coast, arrived in France in 2008 after his studies in Morocco. He and his future wife Ama, from Ivory Coast, have many nephews at home. He declared that his parents told him: "When will you give us our grandchildren? We want to cuddle them before we die." As for Ama, she states:

> When my father says over the phone, "The great and true treasure is your children, not the children of your brothers or sisters. For me, my treasure is you, my children. So, if you want to have your wealth later, you must have your own children. It's they who will take care of you later, not your brothers' children or your sisters' children".

After that, Ama hangs up the phone and cries.

For married couples, infertility is an overwhelming experience in a context of migration as well as in Africa (Duchesne, 2016). Infertility and treatment-seeking are never randomly disclosed and are usually kept secret from people who play no role in the process. Generally, access to ART must remain secret from the close family and the collateral relatives (sisters, brothers or cousins). Only specific key people were involved in treatment procedures and these were part of the patients' trusted circle.

Obtaining reproductive care

The way African people experience and deal with infertility is strongly related to their socio-cultural and economic life circumstances as well as to the availability and non-availability of healthcare options (Gerrits and Shaw, 2010). The quest for conception is nothing new for women in Africa. They are used to moving away from their homes to seek to conceive: to visit a sacred place or a sanctuary to carry out therapeutic rituals (Journet, 1981), to consult various Muslim doctors or *marabouts* or faith healers who belong to specific churches, to visit specific healers (who treat with plants or mineral and animal products), herbalists or "traditional" practitioners (Sundby, 2002; Hörbst, 2006). In rural areas, as in urban areas, in vitro fertilisation (IVF) is usually seen as an extreme option, to be chosen only as a last resort, based on a doctor's prescription.

Also in France, the women interviewed are the first to consult a specialist. Generally they consulted in private centres, seeing several gynaecologists in the course of their search. In fact they do not know how to choose a specialist, and their husband cannot help them. Even in France, infertile couples seek religious support to optimise their chances: they go on a pilgrimage (for example to Lourdes), to an evangelical church or Muslim prayers. A few women also obtain from their own country natural medicines believed to increase fertility. Sometimes a woman consulted at the same time in a private clinic and in a public hospital, to optimise her chances of success.

Since the 1980s, ART procedures have been offered at clinics in sub-Saharan Africa, albeit on a very small scale (Feldman-Savelsberg, 2002). For example, it is relatively well known that the first IVF birth was in 1984 in South Africa, 1989 in Nigeria, 1997 in Togo, 1998 in Cameroon, 2000 in Mali, 2005 in Mauritania, and 2006 in Kenya. In many African countries, actors do not always agree on a single date, because of the challenges of competition in the private ART arena (Bonnet, 2016). Most private clinics offering ART are based in capital cities. In African countries where ART has been introduced, its use has preceded regulation and legislation. Clinics do not need accreditation and neither national legislation nor ethics committees regulate the use of ART in sub-Saharan countries. Several sub-Saharan African ART centres collaborate with ART centres in Europe, the USA, Australia and/or South Africa – where many of the doctors implementing ART received their training (Hörbst, 2012a).

Various forms of ART are offered, in particular artificial insemination using the husband's sperm (AI), donor insemination (DI) and IVF. A few countries, such as Cameroon, Ghana, Nigeria, South Africa and Zimbabwe, also offer other techniques, such as intracytoplasmic sperm injection (ICSI) and embryo freezing. In a few cases the use of donor material – semen, egg and embryos – is also reported. The costs of ART vary considerably from place to place. For instance, the cost of ART in 2012 in Ivory Coast was between 2 million and 3 million CFA francs (i.e. between 3,000–4,000 euros), according to women's age, sperm quality and various other parameters. The high costs of ART compared to the average local income, in combination with the lack of state support and health insurance covering these expenses, make ART unaffordable and inaccessible for the average sub-Saharan African citizen (Donkor and Sandall, 2007).

Those who have opted for cross-border reproductive care, after using several healers and practitioners in their home country, belong to the new African middle class (Darmon, 2012) that contrasts with the very economically vulnerable class living in rural areas. Most often ART is not possible and not available in their country (for example, in Guinea or in Comoros). They have to arrange travel and schedule the consultations themselves, using word-of-mouth advice and help from their informal networks. Patients with family living in France used these contacts for support, both to identify the best "doctor" (gynaecologist) for treatment and to obtain accommodation during their stay in France.

Women's experiences of reproductive mobility

Transnational movements of people with reproductive motivations have developed inside the well-known "reproscape" (Inhorn and Patricio, 2009). Some travel takes place inside Africa, for example from Gabon to Cameroon (Central Africa), or from Guinea to Senegal (West Africa) or from Mozambique to South Africa (Southern Africa); other movements are from Africa to Europe, but also from America to Africa (Cameroon), or from Europe (France) to Africa (Ghana). People may also travel between several places around the world: for example, Mrs Binour, who lives and works in Comoros, went first to Malaysia and then to Egypt, and was consulting in the French physician's office when I met her.

We often forget that biomedical actors, such as secretaries, have to communicate by phone with persons from abroad when booking appointments and also for the start of the process before the arrival in France. In a physician's office (Seine-Saint-Denis, December 2012), the secretary is on the phone with a man calling from Gabon: "IVF and insemination are not the same! We need your serology, sir." It is not sufficient to speak French to ensure mutual understanding (choice of words and accent) and secretaries are not familiar with the economic and health context of African countries. Yet most African people are not familiar with biomedical vocabulary, especially in the beginning.

Despite having a general idea of what procedures they were going through each time, women patients' knowledge about what was happening inside their bodies was rather vague. The use of medical jargon and the French language consultations contribute to the limited perception of treatment. Communication in French may pose a significant barrier to some patients' understanding, leading to anxiety. All the women preferred to see a nurse (working in the private sector) to ensure ovarian stimulation treatment was correctly administered at home. Except for one woman, they were not at all familiar with biomedicine practices.

Accessing IVF services, whether private or public, in France is a heavy economic burden for African couples living in an African country. They use multiple strategies to raise the funds they need for treatment abroad, including saving money over a period of time, taking out bank loans (normally "multipurpose" loans for ART and other expenses), selling personal assets (when extended families had "extra" assets such as real estate, they sold them to pay for treatments), and/or using extra income from collective funding schemes (Bonnet and Duchesne, 2014). The amount spent on treatments was considerable, and the initial budget would often be exceeded during the procedure.

Generally, only the women stayed in France during treatment. Two women interviewed stayed with their sisters, and two others stayed with their sisters-in-law. Monique, from Cameroon, had a stillborn baby in 2005 with her first husband. During her annual vacation, she came to France for her first IVF (with ICSI) because analyses showed that her new husband had "a few problems with his sperm". She said:

Before, I had no [infertility problem], not until I remarried. For my husband, it is finished, he gave his ... well, he gave a sample ... and he went back [to Cameroon]. It is not the same for me, because of stimulation.

One brief return visit for sperm collection is enough for husbands, while women have to stay longer for treatments and egg retrieval. Throughout their search for treatment, women activated social networks (family and friends) to obtain support and information. The choice of a specialist or a particular hospital depends on selected friends or a person of trust. These networks helped them in their quest to find a "trusted" gynaecologist (rather than a clinic), as well as with practical issues such as funding and sometimes accommodation in France, and emotional support. Nevertheless, some women can have an overwhelming sense of loneliness.

Conclusion

The advent of ART has raised new ethical, medical and social issues with the apparent increase in people travelling outside their home country to access these techniques. After a fruitful debate about the improper use of the term "reproductive tourism" (Matorras, 2005; Pennings, 2005), finding a name for this phenomenon was a long-debated issue (Hudson et al., 2011). However, the term *cross-border reproductive care* (CBRC) is increasingly used (Gürtin and Inhorn, 2011). CBRC is considered a worldwide and growing phenomenon (Ferraretti et al., 2010; Gürtin and Inhorn, 2011; Rozée, 2011).

These findings on the therapeutic itineraries of infertile African couples have shown how women – or couples – will do whatever they can to achieve their parenthood projects. They highlight the stigmatisation of sterility in sub-Saharan Africa and the political resistance to declaring it a full-fledged public health problem. Infertility also raises the issue of gender relations. It shows how very vulnerable women are in a context where men are reluctant to acknowledge their sterility, despite the fact that physicians regard it as a common condition.

Women develop various strategies to optimise conception in their home country and then in another country where they have relatives: they manage to find considerable sums of money, and multiply ART care in different clinics or hospitals. They use ART in vulnerable conditions: an unfamiliar environment (a foreign country, unknown medical arena), secret and private environment (with confidence and emotional support only from very close family – often collateral relatives); loneliness (far from the husband and the rest of the family and friends); stigmatisation (because of childlessness or having only one daughter), all of which may lead to distress. On the one hand, it is possible for infertile couples to access new therapeutic options such as ART in private clinics in Africa or elsewhere. On the other hand, these African experiences reveal how structural inequalities are reproduced through healthcare privatisation and the role of global capitalism. Crossing borders in order to conceive a child with biomedical assistance also has many social and psychological impacts. For women in particular, such a transnational pathway could be a perpetual race forward which keeps them on the move, with no guarantee of finally having a child. Notably, CBRC may take the form of (biomedical) roaming.

Notes

1 From 1905 to 1958, French Equatorial Africa was a French-governed federation that included the present-day states of Chad, the Central African Republic, Republic of the Congo and Gabon.
2 Website: www.amp.hypotheses.org. A collective publication is in press.
3 Acknowledgements: I am deeply grateful to the staff of the ART consultations in Paris and in Noisy-le-Grand whose help was crucial to the development of my fieldwork. I am also deeply obliged to the women and to the men who shared with me their reproductive histories and concerns about founding a family, and without whom this research would have neither subject nor purpose.
4 The misnamed "bride price" is in fact "a counter gift" for the wife's fertility (Duchesne, 2014).

References

Boerma, J.T., Mgalla, Z. (eds). 2001. *Women and infertility in sub-Saharan Africa: A multi-disciplinary perspective*, Amsterdam, The Netherlands, KIT.

Bonnet, D. 2014. Adopter un enfant dans le contexte de l'assistance médicale à la procréation en Afrique subsaharienne, *Cahiers d'Etudes Africaines*, LIV 215(3):769–786.

Bonnet, D. 2016. L'assistance médicale à la procréation en Afrique subsaharienne est-elle une innovation sociale? In Haxaire C., Moutaud, B., Farnarier, C. (eds), *L'innovation en santé. Technologie, organisation, changement*, Rennes, Presses Universitaires de Rennes.

Bonnet, D., Duchesne, V. 2014. Migrer pour procréer. Histoires de couples africains [Migrating to procreate: tales of African couples], *Cahiers du Genre*, special issue "Biotechnologies et travail reproductif. Une perspective transnationale [Biotechnologies and Reproductive Work. A transnational Perspective]", 56:41–58

Cooper, B. 2013. De quoi la crise démographique au Sahel est-elle le nom?, *Politique Africaine*, 2(130):69–88.

Darmon, D. 2012. Classes moyennes: une revue de la littérature. Un concept utile pour suivre les dynamiques de l'Afrique, *Afrique Contemporaine*, 4(244):33–51.

Donkor, S., Sandall, J. 2007. The impact of perceived stigma and mediating social factors on infertility-related stress among women seeking infertility treatment in Southern Ghana, *Social Science & Medicine*, 65:1683–1694.

Duchesne, V. 1998. Gémellité, fécondité et souveraineté chez les Anyi de Côte d'Ivoire, *L'UOMO*, 1:137–155.

Duchesne, V. 2014. Repenser l'alliance matrimoniale avec l'AMP en situation migratoire, *Enfances, Familles, Générations*, 21:135–149.

Duchesne, V. 2016. Des corps reproducteurs féminins sous surveillance. Téléphonie mobile et assistance médicale à la procréation dans le contexte de familles africaines transnationales, In Haxaire, C., Moutaud, B., Farnarier, C. (eds), *L'innovation en santé. Technologie, organisation, changement,* Rennes, Presses Universitaires de Rennes.

Dyer, S., Abrahams, N., Mokoena, N., Van Der Spuy, Z.M. 2004. "You are a man because you have children": Experiences, reproductive health knowledge and treatment seeking behaviour among men suffering from couple infertility in South Africa, *Human Reproduction*, 19:960–967.

Ericksen, K., Brunette, T. 1996. Patterns and predictors of infertility among African women: A cross-national survey of twenty-seven nations, *Social Science and Medicine*, 42(2):209–220.

Feldman-Savelsberg, P. 2002. Is infertility an unrecognized public health and population problem? The view from the Cameroon grassfields, in Inhorn, M.C., van Balen, F. (eds), *Infertility around the globe. New thinking on childlessness, gender, and reproductive technologies*, Berkeley & Los Angeles, California, University of California Press: 215–232.

Ferraretti, A.P., Pennings, G., Gianaroli, L., Natali, F., Magli, M.C. 2010. Cross-border reproductive care: a phenomenon expressing the controversial aspects of reproductive technologies, *Reproductive Biomedicine Online*, 20:261–266.

Gerrits, T., Shaw, M. 2010. Biomedical infertility care in sub-Saharan Africa: A social science review of current practices, experiences and viewpoints, *FV&V in ObGyn*, 2 (3):194–207.

Gürtin, Z., Inhorn, M. 2011. Introduction: Travelling for conception and the global assisted reproduction market, *Reproductive Biomedicine Online*, 23(5):535–537.

Hörbst, V. 2006. Infertility and In-vitro Fertilization in Bamako, Mali: Women's experience, Avenues for Solution and Social Contexts Impacting on Gynaecological Consultations, *Curare*, 29(1):35–46.

Hörbst, V. 2008. Male infertility in Mali: Kinship and impacts on biomedical practice in Bamako, in Brockopp, J., Eich, T. (eds), *Muslim medical ethics: theory and practice*, South Carolina, South Carolina University Press: 118–137.

Hörbst, V. 2012a. Assisted reproduction in Mali and Togo: Circulating knowledge, mobile technology, transnational efforts, in Dilger, H., Kane, A., Langwick, S. (eds), *Transnational medicine, mobile experts: Globalization, health and power in and beyond Africa*, Indiana, Indiana University Press: 163–189.

Hörbst, V. 2012b. 'You need someone in a grand boubou' – barriers and means to access ART in West Africa, *FV&V in ObGyn Monograph*, 46–52.

Hudson, N., Culley, L., Blyth, E., Norton, W., Rapport, F., Pacey, A. 2011. Cross-border reproductive care: A review of the literature, *Reproductive Biomedicine Online*, 22:673–685.

Inhorn, M. C. 2009. Right to assisted reproductive technology: overcoming infertility in low-resource countries, *International Journal of Gynecology and Obstetrics*, 106(2):172–174.

Inhorn, M. 2011. Globalization and gametes: reproductive 'tourism', Islamic bioethics, and Middle Eastern modernity, *Anthropology & Medicine*, 18(1):87–103.

Inhorn M.C., Patricio, P. 2009. Rethinking reproductive "tourism" as reproductive "exile", *Fertility & Sterility*, 92:904–906.

Journet, O. 1981. La quête de l'enfant. Représentation de la maternité et rituels de stérilité dans la société Diola de Basse Casamance, *Journal des Africanistes*, 51(1–2):97–115.

Kamba, M., Tillard, B. 2013. Le fosterage à l'épreuve de la migration. Jeunes Bamiléké du Cameroun accueillis en France, *Ethnologie Française*, 2(43):325–334.

Leonard, L. 2002. Problematizing fertility. "Scientific" accounts and Chadian women's narratives, in Inhorn, M.C., van Balen, F. (eds), *Infertility around the globe. New thinking on childlessness, gender, and reproductive technologies*, Berkeley & Los Angeles, California, University of California Press: 193–215.

Matorras, R. 2005. Reproductive exile versus reproductive tourism, *Human Reproduction*, 20:3,571.

Pennings, G. 2005. Reply: Reproductive exile versus reproductive tourism, *Human Reproduction*, 20:3,571–3,573.

Retel-Laurentin, A. 1974. *Infécondité en Afrique noire. Maladies et conséquences sociales*, Paris, Masson et Cie.

Rozée, V. 2011. L'AMP sans frontière, *Bulletin Epidémiologique Hebdomadaire*, 23–24:270–273.

Rutstein, S.O., Shah, I.H. 2004. *Infecundity, infertility, and childlessness in developing countries*, Calverton, Maryland, ORC Macros/WHO/Measure DHS, Comparative reports, n° 9, p. xiii.

Schuster, S., Hörbst, V. 2006. Introduction. Reproductive disruptions: African perspectives, *Curare*, 29:5–16.

Sundby, J. 2002. Infertility and health care in countries with less resources. Case studies with sub-Saharan Africa, in Inhorn, M.C., van Balen, F. (eds), *Infertility around the globe. New thinking on childlessness, gender, and reproductive technologies*, Berkeley & Los Angeles, California, University of California Press: 247–259.

Tichit, C. 2009. Le spectre de la stérilité en Afrique Centrale, de la question épidémiologique au risque social, in Gourbin, C. (ed.), *Santé de la reproduction au Nord et au Sud. De la connaissance à l'action*, UCL Presses universitaires de Louvain, 257–275.

7 Egg freezing

Portraying a new reproductive technology in the Israeli media

Daphna Birenbaum-Carmeli

The context: Israel's reproductive landscape

Israeli society is family-centered. Despite some erosion of the traditional family, nearly all Jewish and Arab Israelis live in nuclear families (90%). The vast majority of Israeli couples (95%) get married. They do so at a relatively young age (roughly 26)[1] and raise their children together. Eighty-eight per cent of Israeli children up to age 17 live with their two parents.[2] By the age of 65, only 3% of Israelis have never been married.[3] Very few families – a mere 6% – are single-parented. Of these, only 15% are headed by a never-married woman; this low percentage is nonetheless roughly twice that of 2000.[4]

Personal status, including marriage, paternity and divorce, are all regulated by religious courts, each ruling its own community. Civil marriage is prohibited and inter-religious marriage, which requires conversion of one spouse, is extremely rare.

With a total fertility rate of 3.03,[5] Israeli women bear twice as many children as their EU counterparts (1.56)[6] and 50% more than American women (2.01).[7] Women's age at first childbirth has risen, but remains relatively low at 27 years.[8]

Jewish Israeli familism has commonly been traced to religious and political sources. Placing the Biblical commandment "be fruitful and multiply" center stage, childbearing merges the private and the political (Swirski 1976:129–130), comprising a pivot in the mature life of Jewish persons and their contribution to the collectivity's regeneration (e.g. Gold 1988:23–27; Safir 1991). The traumas of the Holocaust and immigration, alongside demographic politics, further enhance the significance of procreation as a cornerstone of the nation's construction (Teman 2003). The majority of Israelis agree that "childless people live an empty life" (56%) and nearly all (90%) accept that "raising one's children is life's greatest joy" (Glickman 2003). Taxation and labor laws are pronatalist, though, to a fairly moderate extent (Birenbaum-Carmeli and Carmeli 2010).

In vitro fertilization (IVF) was introduced to Israel relatively early, in 1981. The technology quickly spread, making Israeli women its heaviest consumers (Birenbaum-Carmeli 1997, forthcoming; Collins 2002). Medical professionals, service providers, politicians, religious authorities as well as lay persons and feminists all welcomed IVF, approving multiple uses without ever seriously questioning their implications.

The state's role in this warm acceptance was decisive, when it set a policy of universal, publicly funded IVF to all Israeli woman aged 18 to 45, irrespective of sexual orientation or psychological, financial or family status, up to the birth of two live children with the woman's current partner, if applicable. The state also entitles IVF "patients" to 20 days' sick-leave for each IVF cycle and protects them from being fired while on treatment. Between 1990 and 2012, the rate of IVF cycles per 1,000 mounted from 4.5 to the world's highest rate of 21.0.[9] Given the major crisis in Israel's public healthcare, and the complete lack of state support for adoption (Birenbaum-Carmeli and Carmeli 2010),[10] the expansive IVF policy underscores the weight of biogenetic filiality as a state priority.

Israelis appear to share the state's preference for biogenetic over social relatedness. Until the mid-1990s, male infertility was practically intractable. Heterosexual couples who made use of donor sperm tended to ask gynecologists for a donor who resembled the intended father and hid the donor insemination from their surroundings (Birenbaum-Carmeli, Carmeli and Yavetz 2000; Birenbaum-Carmeli, Carmeli and Cohen 2000). In later years, when IVF became routinized, it spread throughout all social strata in Israel, marginalizing all alternatives to family formation. Women who were undergoing IVF never even considered any other option and were unrealistically optimistic regarding the chance of treatment success. At the same time, women tended to downplay concomitant risks as well as the overall impact of repeated IVF cycles on their lives, careers and economic situations. When asked – in an open question – how many IVF cycles they would be willing to undergo, the vast majority of the women (87%) replied "as many as needed" (Birenbaum-Carmeli and Dirnfeld 2008).

Similar determination regarding conception can be witnessed in other modes of conception that Israelis undertake. Egg donations are extremely rare in Israel. Women and couples who require donor eggs, therefore, travel abroad or else contact Israeli doctors who have established connections with egg donors in foreign countries, in order to obtain such eggs. This road to family formation entails high costs and complicated logistics but is nonetheless very popular.

Gay individuals and couples are not eligible for egg donation and surrogacy in Israel. Consequently, numerous gay Israelis undertake cross-border gestational surrogacy in order to found genetically related families. More than any other, this form of ART requires extreme investment in terms of time, logistics and money, which amount to the price of an apartment in Israel. Still, hundreds of Israeli gay men pursue this road to parenthood. Moreover, most of these Israelis go on and attempt to have more than one child, i.e. found a "full family" in local terms, rather than raise a single child. To supplement these examples that illustrate the extent of effort and monetary investment that Israeli individuals and couples are willing to make in pursuit of parenthood and family, one could look at the exceptional hostility that is directed at the few Israelis who choose to remain voluntarily childless (Donath 2010).

Egg freezing by vitrification

Though various attempts to freeze human ova have taken place since the 1980s, and though the first baby was born from a frozen egg in 1986 (Lockwood 2011), previous methods were relatively ineffective (de Melo-Martin and Cholst 2008). The method at hand, "egg vitrification", is a form of flash freezing that has proved more efficient, enabling more eggs to thaw viably (Lockwood 2011). In the present chapter, I use the terms "vitrification" and "freezing" interchangeably. Like its predecessors, egg vitrification starts as a regular IVF cycle, namely by hormone stimulation of the woman's ovaries, aiming to induce the maturation of numerous follicles, followed by surgical aspiration of the mature follicles. In a regular IVF cycle, the follicles are placed in a petri dish with ejaculated sperm to fertilize in an incubator. When the egg is about to be vitrified, it is transferred to the laboratory for flash freezing.

Egg vitrification is the newest addition to Israel's expansive ART palette. This novel method of flash freezing can potentially prolong women's reproductive life-span by storing eggs of women in their 20s and 30s for later use, when the woman is in her 40s and even later in life (Goold and Savulescu 2009; Shkedi-Rafid and Hashiloni-Dolev 2012).

Egg vitrification was introduced to Israel in the past decade (Mertes and Pennings 2012). As of 2011, Ministry of Health (MoH) regulations allow the use of the technology also for social reasons (Shkedi-Rafid and Hashiloni-Dolev 2011, 2012; Stoop 2010). In October 2012, the American Society for Reproductive Medicine lifted the experimental ban on the technology and approved its use also for "social" reasons in the United States (Lunau 2012; Nicefaro 2012; Richards 2012).

Since the 2011 approval of Israel's MoH, local IVF clinics have invited women to have their own eggs frozen. Two major subpopulations are interested in the new service: 1) *medical:* women diagnosed with cancer whose treatment may harm their ovarian function, or women at risk of premature menopause; 2) *social:* mostly single women who, for educational, career, economic or relational reasons, are concerned about "aging out" of their fertility (Mertes and Pennings 2012; Stoop, Nekkebroeck and Devroey 2011). Women belonging to the first category are entitled to free service, covered by Israel's National Health Insurance. Women from the latter category have to fund the treatment – 3,000–8,000 USD – out of their own pocket. Women are allowed to undergo up to four treatment cycles, or until they have 20 eggs frozen. Women are allowed to have the cryopreserved eggs thawed, fertilized and transferred back to the uterus until they are 54 years of age. Women are required to sign a declaration confirming that they are aware that the treatment provides no guarantee of future conception (Geva 2011).

Very little information is available regarding the women who endorse egg vitrification, especially for "social" reasons; in the United States, a preliminary study reported women's average age as 38. From their own descriptions, the women emerge as highly educated, intelligent, extroverted and single, desiring to release the pressure of aging while they search for a suitable partner (Gold et al. 2006).

In Israel, preliminary findings (Birenbaum-Carmeli, forthcoming(a)) suggest a similar profile of the women who undertake egg freezing for "social" reasons: the women are in their later 30s and are highly educated. Most have had a serious relationship that eventually broke up, and are hoping to establish stable relationships and have children. A few mentioned they thought about the frozen eggs for their second child. A study that took place a short while before the approval of the procedure for social reasons revealed that the lay public knows very little about the new technology (Hashiloni-Dolev et al. 2011).

Methodology

Given the scarce knowledge regarding egg vitrification, media presentations of the subject have an especially formative impact on lay perceptions regarding this new option. The present study probes early presentations of the subject in the Hebrew press in the period between 2008 and 2012. The articles were collected via internet search, conducted during the month of December 2013. Articles were retrieved by inserting into a Google search the following terms in Hebrew: "social egg freezing", "social egg preservation" and "egg freezing/preservation procedure". The fifteen scrutinized articles were the first to appear in the search at that point in time. The sources of the articles were diverse and distributed as following: Ten of the articles appeared in the online versions of daily newspapers: *Yedioth – Ynet/Xnet* (5), *Maariv – NRG* (3), *Haaretz* (1), *Israel Hayom* (1) and *Calcalist* (1). The remaining five articles appeared in a parents' magazine (2), a major doctors' website (2) and a popular news website (1). The articles' details are listed at the end of this chapter. The articles' sequential numbers from this list are shown in square brackets to identify each article in the sections below, which elucidate the main themes that emerged from the content analysis.

The media coverage of egg vitrification in Israel

A "rosy" depiction of the technology

The Israeli Hebrew media received egg vitrification with a warm welcome. First, the media established the efficiency of the new technology. An optimistic portrayal highlighted benefits and tended to marginalize potential problems and failures. One article boasted a sensationalizing title: "Mother at any age", heralding "The birth age revolution" [3] by capitalizing on the exemplary story of actress Jennifer Aniston, who had presumably undertaken egg freezing. Another article, in its report of the recent approval of social egg freezing, informed readers that 20 eggs, the maximum number allowed in "social freezing", "are enough, in most cases, to produce several children" [12]. Other articles construed images of success by citing scientific articles that found 80–90% egg survival rates and even beyond [3, 8] and promising pregnancy rates reaching up to 40% and 50% per treatment cycle [3, 8]. One well-known fertility expert reassured the readers that "today, there is no difference in the quality of frozen and fresh eggs" [11]. Within this picture, egg freezing could be presented as an "insurance measure" [16].

The promising depictions were supplemented by presentations of the procedure as simple, straightforward and efficient: "Career women want to delay their fertility. These women simply turn to egg freezing" [14]. "In the future, when the woman wishes to become pregnant, the eggs will be thawed and fertilized with her partner's sperm" [8].

One aspect of the simplifying descriptions was the language of control. Some articles presented egg freezing as a preplanned scheme that could be enacted by the woman at her will and produce the expected result:

> One cannot stop time but thanks to the advancement of medicine, one can try to control it. It is now possible to freeze unfertilized eggs, allowing any woman who wants to, to time her deliveries so they fit into her schedule.
>
> [2]

Technology was thus constituted in this presentation as a counterweight, probably a "remedy", to nature and normal age-related decline in women's fertility. Egg freezing was presented as enabling women to prolong their reproductive years and give birth at any time of their choice. As such, egg freezing was integrated as a new component into Israelis' general faith in technological progress, a consistent disposition observed throughout decades of reproductive technologies in Israel (Birenbaum-Carmeli 1997).

The "rosy" image that journalists drew was manifested also in the use of positive, reassuring vocabulary. They called egg freezing "a lifesaver", cited fertility experts who entitled the technology "Revolutionary" [3], "science fiction" [5] and even "a miracle" [5], and who compared its contribution and impact to those of the pill [3]. The doctors also reassured the readers that older women cope well with pregnancy [5] and glorified older parents as being patient, relaxed and well off economically. At the same time, they marginalized problems that accompanied egg freezing, such as high cost to the consumers, health risks to the woman and, maybe most of all, the uncertainty regarding future conception that the novel, little-known technology actually offered.

To further reinforce the importance of the new technology, the journalists criticized the lack of public funding to social egg freezing as discriminatory and called to instate state coverage for the procedure also for social causes.

Approval on the part of clinicians and religious authorities

Professional and ethical support augmented the image of reliable technology. To that end, clinicians were cited as they were urging women to make use of vitrification. One article quantified the practitioners' endorsement by citing a recent survey that contended that 80% of the directors of IVF units in Israel were supportive of egg vitrification also for social reasons [14]. Another article cited a study that found that the resulting babies were as healthy as any others, maybe even more so [16]. A high level of support, grounded by the specific figure of 81%, was attributed to bioethicists as well [14].

Religious authorities in Israel were depicted as equally positive. Reporters cited rabbis who acknowledged the growing number of religious women who had not married and approved egg freezing in order to enable these women to conceive at a later time in their lives. The following quote was typical:

> We would, obviously, prefer women to give birth when God had intended them to. However, we cannot ignore the agony. Women fail to marry. Therefore, as an interim solution, we support EF. This is certainly preferable to sperm banking, which is religiously forbidden.
>
> [10]

The latter part in the rabbi's opinion refers to the Jewish traditional prohibition on "wasting one's sperm", which applies to sperm banking as well. So much so that several rabbis were cited, in the context of egg vitrification, as comparing the use of donor sperm to prostitution [10, 11]. Donor sperm is, nonetheless, allowed when needed, if the sperm being used is that of a non-Jewish man, which also removes the fear of future incest (Soffer and Birenbaum-Carmeli 2010, Inhorn et al. forthcoming). Juxtaposing the two options to conception that are open to unwed Jewish women who wish to become mothers – using donor sperm to become a single mother or freezing one's eggs for later use, hopefully with a partner – the rabbi made a decisive preference in favor of the latter because it does not require donor sperm. The only concern that rabbis expressed in the media regarding egg freezing was that its availability might relieve women's sense of urgency, which might lead them to wait longer until they marry.

Depicting gendered bodies: images of fertility decline

Inherent in the depiction of egg freezing was the scientific narrative of women's bodily deterioration, which underlies the very need for egg freezing. In a manner somewhat similar to that observed by Emily Martin (1991), the Israeli press underscored women's declining fertility during their 30s:

> It turns out, my dear, that no matter how you look and no matter how young you feel, in matters of reproduction, it is only your age that counts.
>
> [17]

Article writers juxtaposed women's fertility against men's, emphasizing the difference [14]:

> Unlike a man who produces sperm throughout his entire life, women are born with a fixed number of eggs, which decline in number and quality along their lives. A steep decrease starts when the woman is 35–37 and continues beyond age 40 … The older the woman and the longer the freezing, the higher the likelihood that the pregnancy will terminate in miscarriage or impaired fetus.
>
> [2]

Several journalists contended that women were living in denial, refusing to accept the reality of their diminishing fertility and therefore often delayed egg freezing beyond its optimal timing [17].

At the margins of this gendered aspect of the coverage, one should note that among the professionals that were quoted in the press, one lawyer and two senior fertility experts were women. More generally, several articles seemed to try to associate egg freezing with female empowerment. Thus, the lawyer mentioned above, the legal advisor to the MoH, stressed the contribution of egg vitrification to enable women to be "responsible for their reproductive destiny" [3]. Another article presented the technology as narrowing the gender gap, by offering women gamete freezing, an option that men have had for a few decades. "This is part of making women equal to men", a journalist quoted a fertility expert [13].

Another gender issue that appeared on the margins of a few articles was the moral standing of late motherhood. Though it presumably addressed the issue of gender equality, to the best of my recollection, late fatherhood and its moral standing have never been discussed in the Israeli media.

Establishing demand for the procedure

The portrayal of the bodily deterioration was supplemented by a description of women's eagerness to undergo the procedure. One article quoted a doctor who described the numerous phone calls he was receiving regularly from women who were seeking egg freezing [14]. A message of urgency was conveyed also by the story of an Israeli woman who was determined to have her eggs frozen before "social egg freezing" was available in Israel. The woman, aged 40, went to Kiev with an Israeli fertility expert in order to undergo the procedure. The woman, described as a career woman, elucidated how egg freezing improved her life:

> I wanted to make sure that when I wish to have children with a partner, I'll have a chance to do that with my own eggs. This procedure will allow me to conceive at an age when fertility might be problematic ... now I am a more whole person. I stopped fearing the passing time.
>
> [13]

Several messages were implied in the story: i) that bearing genetically related children was superior to socially related ones; ii) that egg freezing provided no guarantee of pregnancy; iii) that a woman aged 40 was still fertile enough to find reassurance in having her own eggs frozen for future use, "when fertility might be problematic". Overall, the story suggested that a woman can conceive and give birth well into her 40s, and possibly, with egg freezing, even later, into the sixth decade of her life. Notably, the article did mention, if only in passing, that prior to the woman's trip to Kiev, she had been refused by five gynecologists whom she requested to help her have her eggs frozen abroad. However, the journalist presented the woman's perseverance with great sympathy and framed the final outcome as a reassuring accomplishment. Similar stories were published when egg vitrification for social reasons became available in Israel [14]. The state policy that approved egg freezing up to the age of 41 augmented the same message regarding the timeline of women's fertility.

The bleak side: depicting complications

The articles were not one-sided, though. Practically each piece of communication included various types of precautions as well. Experts warning from complications like ovarian hyper-stimulations or ovarian torsion were prevalent [e.g. 2, 17], as were references to poorer egg quality in later years [14] and higher risk of pregnancy complications [13, 17]. Since the Israeli policy allows egg freezing to the age of 41 and transplanting the thawed fertilized eggs until the woman turns 54, this aspect of vitrification was especially relevant. Experts also mentioned the lack of clarity regarding the long-term consequences of the procedure which was part of its novelty and the meager available experience. The following reminder, from a fertility expert, a man, was typical:

> This is an experimental technology with a low success rate. We should be careful not to raise false hopes.
>
> [3]

Later on in the article, the doctor acknowledged that there was little experience with pregnancies from vitrified eggs among reproductively older women and that there may be more pregnancy complications and lower rates of success [8]. One article mentioned the length of the freezing time as an unknown factor that needed to be further explored as well as the concern that the freezing materials might be harmful to the future fetus [14]. Several articles called doctors to ensure that the women understood that the procedure did not guarantee a future pregnancy and mentioned the doctors' economic interests in the provision of the privately funded service [14].

One instance of pronounced reservation which the reporters conveyed related to the bar project. Initiated by several fertility experts, including a prominent female gynecologist, this team of clinicians approached women in their 30s who were sitting in bars in the evenings and started a conversation on fertility decline and fertility preservation by means of egg vitrification. According to the press, the experts wanted "to encourage egg freezing during the 30s, among women who do not feel ready to conceive right now" [16]. The journalist added her own opinion that:

> They don't want to know that after 40 it is not really easy to conceive and that after 44 there is hardly any chance at all … because we love to feel young.
>
> [16]

Women's reactions were, however, by and large resentful, rejecting the attempt to educate them while they were out, drinking and enjoying themselves. The women viewed the initiative as intrusive and patronizing, assuming they were ignorant and in denial of the decline in their own fertility. The project was soon discontinued.

Notably, in the 2015 conference of the Israeli Fertility Association, an Israeli expert presented a statistical model in which he estimated that when using eggs frozen when the women was 35, the woman would need 36 eggs for a likelihood of 90% to achieve live birth. If she froze them when she was 40, the respective figure rose to 60 eggs. My search has not revealed any reference to these new figures in any Hebrew channel of communication.

The importance of childbearing: egg freezing as "second best"

Underlying the favorable depiction of egg vitrification was the assumption regarding childbearing as crucial to one's happiness and self-accomplishment. The message was focused, more specifically, on women rather than on couples and families, stressing that women who did not marry also deserved to bear their own children. Egg freezing was thus constituted as a "second best", a suboptimal option to be undertaken when the more desirable alternative of normative family seemed to be fading out. The words of the legal advisor of the [MoH], a woman, when announcing the approval of egg freezing for social reasons, were instructive:

> I don't expect masses of women to seek egg vitrification. At the end of the day, every woman aspires to establish couplehood and conceive naturally.
>
> [12]

The superiority of the natural course of conception was reasserted repeatedly:

> The procedure [egg freezing] does not guarantee a pregnancy at the end of the road ... It is therefore recommended, despite the technological progress, to include family planning at the proper age rather than postpone it to very late in women's lives.
>
> [2]

A similar message was embedded in the press portrayal of the female clientele as accomplished women in their 30s, all single:

> These are accomplished, successful singles, many of them are religious women who acquired high education, made a career; they are thoroughly self-actualized and the gap between them and most men makes it harder to find a partner ... [However, there are also] numerous women who are as far from religion as they are from the moon. Some are even anti-religious, and they all want families and children, and they all prefer to have the baby with a father rather than from an anonymous sperm donor.
>
> [11]

Doctors subscribed to this perception as well. In one article, an expert was cited saying: "I wouldn't recommend it to a married career woman" [3], thereby distinguishing – an evidently non-medical distinction – between "justified" and "less justified" social causes for egg freezing. According to this hierarchy, absence of a partner was an acceptable cause for pregnancy postponement and egg freezing, whereas a woman's career was not. These depictions all conveyed a similar message: that beyond their variability, all Israeli women, accomplished and professionally successful as they may be, wish to have children, preferably within a traditional two-parent family. Egg freezing was thus presented as a means to help women found traditional, heteronormative families rather than resort to single motherhood.

Nationalist aspect

Still broader was the argument, or rather the context-specific feature, of nationalism, as applied to childbearing. Journalists emphasized the crucial importance of childbearing in the Israeli context: "for us [Israelis], there is only one type of *Nachat* [happiness from one's children]: grandchildren" [16]. In one article, the legal advisor to the MoH, a woman, explicitly represented the state administration, promising that "the state of Israel is set and ready to help any woman to bear children" [12]. In another article, the speaker linked this heightened importance of childbearing to the Jewish history, contending that:

> We are different – a people who underwent holocaust is unlike any other in terms of attitude to family and continuity. In Norway, a mother, a father and a dog is fine while a mother and a father with two children are a phenomenon. For us, the yearning for family and continuity ... is very strong, and I identify with this completely.
>
> [11]

The speakers thus framed egg vitrification in a broad, national context, invoking the deep seated link between one's own children and the collective quest to reproduce the Jewish people. Again, ARTs were constituted as an auxiliary to accomplishing personal as well as collective goals.

Discussion

The Israeli popular press introduced the new technology of egg vitrification primarily favorably, portraying a practical solution to aging for women in their late 30s who wished to bear genetically related offspring at some point in the future. The vocabulary, the personal stories, the doctors' quotations were by and large in favor of the recent innovation. The state policy was, obviously, a major component in the positive framing, as it granted egg freezing the seal of state approval. The media was not, however, one-sided. Practically every article mentioned above clarified that freezing one's eggs was not a guarantee of future conception and that pregnancies at a later age had a higher rate of complications. Both aspects of the coverage, the supportive and the more reluctant, however, reaffirmed the centrality of childbearing for Israeli women, the superiority of biogenetic over social relatedness and of the two-parent family over that of a single mother. The coverage seemed then to try and sustain both ends: elicit women's hopes and faith in egg freezing, while mentioning, if more marginally, the technology's shortcomings, so as to provide a realistic and fair depiction and keep women's hopes within probable range.

The social issues that were embedded in egg vitrification were hardly addressed. Probably the most prominent in this silenced category was that of the struggle of contemporary women to balance work and family life within the confines of the biological life cycle. Only one article addressed this difficulty and included a doctor's reservation regarding the medical solution of what he considered a social problem: "It is shocking and scary to find out that the medical solution is accepted so easily" [14].

In this respect, too, egg freezing, which was heralded as a reproductive revolution, seems to be smoothly incorporated into existing, traditional perceptions and power relations that have been governing family and reproduction in Israel for decades.

List of press sources

1   Solomon, S. We haven't missed the train yet. *Parents and Children Magazine.* December 25, 2011.
2   Doctors. Egg Freezing: Fertility Preservation. *Doctors.* February 16, 2012.
3   Yasour Beit-Or, M. From this day on: Every woman aged 30–41 will be able to freeze eggs. *Mothers at every age.* January 18, 2011.
4   Sheffer, H. Calcalist reviews: A market for the rich only: What is left from the message about Egg Freezing? *Calcalist.* January 12, 2011.
5   Shperling, N. Egg Freezing: Not what you had in mind. *Doctors.* July 11, 2011.
6   A report: Jennifer Aniston is pregnant. Lifestyle, *Ynet.* May 15, 2015.
7   Shnaid, O. The next frozen thing. *Parents and Children.* February 21, 2008.
8   Elitzur, S. To stop the biological clock: Egg Freezing. *NRG, Maariv.* November 30, 2011.
9   Fatwa: Unmarrieds are allowed to freeze eggs. *Only good things.* December 19, 2010.
10 Bashan, T. The fertility revolution: 4 women who froze eggs are talking for the first time. *Nrg, Maariv.* January 14, 2011.
11 Gal, I. Health Ministry Approved: Egg Freezing for Every Woman. On the way to Parenting, *Ynet.* September 6, 2010.
12 Reznik, R. Exposure: Froze eggs and will give birth at her "free time". Frozen Baby, *Ynet.* September 9, 2009.
13 Shir-Raz, Y. Investigation: Is Egg Freezing a Dangerous Illusion? *Ynet.* September 23, 2011.
14 Even, D. Permission was given to woman in Israel to freeze eggs, from career considerations also. *Haaretz.* January 18, 2011.
15 Geva, E. Following the new law: How can you freeze eggs and what is the cost? *Ynet.* January 20, 2011.
16 Lapid, L. "When I'm in the Bar, I don't want to hear I'm getting old". *Xnet.* July 27, 2012.

Notes

1 CSB, Marriages-Selected Data, 2012 figure, http://www.cbs.gov.il/www/population/marrige_divorce/marriage_all.pdf
2 http://www.children.org.il/Files/File/SHNATON/%20%202013.pdf, http://www.cbs.gov.il/reader/newhodaot/hodaa_template.html?hodaa=201511039
3 http://www.cbs.gov.il/shnaton65/st02_04x.pdf
4 http://www.cbs.gov.il/reader/newhodaot/hodaa_template.html?hodaa=201511039
5 http://www.cbs.gov.il/reader/shnaton/templ_shnaton.html?num_tab=st03_13&CYear=2014
6 http://ec.europa.eu/eurostat/tgm/table.do?tab=table&init=1&language=en&pcode=tsdde220&plugin=1
7 https://www.cia.gov/library/publications/the-world-factbook/rankorder/2127rank.html
8 http://www.cbs.gov.il/www/publications/lidot/lidot_table2_11.pdf
9 http://www.health.gov.il/PublicationsFiles/IVF1986_2012.pdf
10 In contrast to the rise in IVF, fewer children are being adopted, e.g. 221 in 2007 vs 88 in 2012.

References

Birenbaum-Carmeli, Daphna. 1997. Pioneering Procreation: Israel's First Test-Tube Baby. *Science as Culture* 6:525–540.

Birenbaum-Carmeli, Daphna. Forthcoming. Thirty Years of ART in Israel. *Reproductive BioMedicine and Society Online*.

Birenbaum-Carmeli, Daphna and Martha Dirnfeld. 2008. The more the better? IVF policy in Israel and women's views. *Reproductive Health matters* 16(31):1–10.

Birenbaum-Carmeli and Yoram S. Carmeli. 2010. Introduction: Reproductive Technologies among Jewish Israelis: Setting the Ground, in D. Birenbaum-Carmeli and Yoram S. Carmeli (eds), *Kin, Gene, Community: Reproductive Technology among Jewish Israelis*, Oxford and New York: Berghahn Books, 1–48.

Birenbaum-Carmeli, Daphna, Yoram S. Carmeli and H. Yavetz. 2000. Secrecy among Israeli recipients of donor insemination. *Politics and the Life Sciences* 19(1):69–76.

Birenbaum-Carmeli, Daphna, Yoram S. Carmeli and Rina Cohen. 2000. Our first 'IVF baby': Israel's and Canada's Press coverage of procreative technology. *International Journal of Sociology and Social Policy* 20(7):1–38.

Collins, J.A. 2002. An International Survey of the Health Economics of IVF and ICSI. *Human Reproductive Update* 8:265–77.

de Melo-Martin, Inmaculada and Ina N. Cholst. 2008. Researching Human Oocyte Cryopreservation: Ethical Issues. *Fertility and Sterility* 89:523–528.

Donath, Orna. 2010. *Making a Choice: Being Childfree in Israel*. Tel Avvi: Yedioth Books.

Geva, E. 2011. Following the new law: How can you Freeze Eggs and what is the cost? *Ynet*. January 20, 2011.

Glickman, A. 2003. Marriage in Israel on the threshold of the 21st century [Hebrew]. *Public Opinion [De'ot Ba'am]*, no. 7.

Gold, E., K. Copperman, G. Witkin, C. Jones and A.B. Copperman. 2006. A Motivational Assessment of Women Undergoing Elective Freezing for Fertility Preservation. *Fertility and Sterility* S201:P–187.

Gold, M. 1988. *And Hannah Wept: Infertility, Adoption and the Jewish Couple*. Philadelphia: The Jewish Publication Society.

Goold, Imogen and Julian Savulescu. 2009. In Favour of Freezing Eggs for Non-medical Reasons. *Bioethics* 23:47–58.

Hashiloni-Dolev, Yael, Amit Kaplan and Shiri Shkedi-Rafid. 2011. The Fertility Myth: Israeli Students' Knowledge Regarding Age-related Fertility Decline and Late Pregnancies in an Era of Assisted Reproduction Technology. *Human Reproduction* 26:3,045–3,053.

Inhorn, Marcia, Birenbaum-Carmeli, Daphna, Soraya Tremayne and Zeynep Gurtin. (Forthcoming). Kinship and Assisted Reproductive Technologies in the Middle East, *The Cambridge Handbook for The Anthropology of Kinship*.

Lockwood, Gillian M. 2011. Social Egg Freezing: The Prospect of Reproductive 'Immortality' or a Dangerous Delusion? *Reproductive BioMedicine Online* 23:334–340.

Lunau, Kate. 2012. Thirty-seven and Counting. *Maclean's* 125:46–50.

Martin, Emily. 1991. The Egg and the Sperm: How Science Has Constructed a Romance Based on Stereotypical Male-Female Roles. *Signs* 16(3):485–501.

Mertes, Heidi and Guido Pennings. 2012. Elective Oocyte Cryopreservation: Who Should Pay? *Human Reproduction* 27:9–13.

Nicefaro, Melissa. 2012. Turning Back the Clock: New Science Helps Older Women Become First-time Mothers. *New Haven Magazine* December:11–39.

Richards, Sarah Elizabeth. 2012. We Need to Talk About Our Eggs. *The New York Times* Oct. 23:A23.

Safir, P. Marilyn. 1991. Religion, Tradition and Public Policy Give Family First Priority, in Swirski Barbara and Marilyn P. Safir (eds), *Calling the Equality Bluff*, New York: Pergamon, 57–65.

Shkedi-Rafid, Shiri and Yael Hashiloni-Dolev. 2011. Egg Freezing for Age-related Fertility Decline: Preventive Medicine or a Further Medicalization of Reproduction? Analyzing the New Israeli Policy. *Fertility and Sterility* 96:291–294.

Shkedi-Rafid, Shiri and Yael Hashiloni-Dolev. 2012. Egg Freezing for Non-medical Uses: The Lack of a Relational Approach to Autonomy in the New Israeli Policy and in Academic Discussion. *Journal of Medical Ethics* 38:154–157.

Soffer, Yigal and D. Birenbaum-Carmeli. 2010. Le don de sperme en Israël ; son secret et son anonymat. *Andrologie: Journal officiel de la Société d'andrologie de langue Française*.

Stoop, Dominic. 2010. Social Oocyte Freezing. *Facts Views & Visions in ObGyn* 2:31–34.

Stoop, D., J. Nekkebroeck and P. Devroey. 2011. A Survey on the Intentions and Attitudes towards Oocyte Cryopreservation for Non-medical Reasons among Women of Reproductive Age. *Human Reproduction* 26:655–661.

Swirski, S. 1976. Community and the Meaning of the Modern State: The Case of Israel. *The Jewish Journal of Sociology* 18:123–40.

Teman, E. 2003. The medicalization of "nature" in the "artificial body": Surrogate motherhood in Israel. *Medical Anthropology Quarterly* 17(1):78–98.

Part II
Surrogacy
Realities and controversies

8   Surrogacy in India

The good, the bad and the ugly

Duru Shah, Sabahat Rasool &
Nagadeepti Nagarajan

The word 'surrogate' literally means 'substitute'. A surrogate mother is therefore a 'substitute mother'. She is a woman who, for financial and/or compassionate reasons, agrees to bear a child for another woman who is unable to or, rarely, unwilling to do so herself. In other words, she is a substitute or 'tentative' mother, in that she conceives, gestates and delivers a baby on behalf of another woman who is subsequently to be seen as the social and legal mother of the child, as has been described by van Niekerk and van Zyl (1995). 'The intended parents', also referred to as 'the commissioning parents' or 'the commissioning couple', is the term used for the couple who intends to extend their family through surrogacy.

Background

Surrogacy in ancient times

Surrogacy can be dated back to Biblical and prehistoric times. The Old Testament (Genesis 16.1–15) records three events of surrogacy, and it appears that the use of a surrogate to circumvent female infertility was an accepted practice in the ancient Far East. One of the incidents mentioned is that of Sarah, who was unable to bear Abraham a child. She told Abraham: 'Behold now, the Lord has prevented me from bearing children; go in to my maid; it may be that I shall obtain children by her.' Abraham did as he was told and, at the age of 90 years, he was able to father a child by Hagar, and Ishmael was born. This clearly depicts that surrogacy has been used since time immemorial to help women who cannot bear children themselves, as stated by Brinsden (2003). Another example from pre-Mosaic times is Jacob bearing children with Leah's maid, Zilpah, on Leah's behalf and with Rachel's maid, Bilhah, on Rachel's behalf. Surrogacy has also been mentioned in Hindu epics like the *Mahabharata*.

Indications for surrogacy by the American Society of Reproductive Medicine (ASRM, 2012) include:

- Women born with no uterus or abnormalities in uterus
- Women who have undergone hysterectomy but have functioning ovaries
- Medical indications contraindicating pregnancy
- Single parent or same-sex couple.

There is no consensus for other indications like repeated IVF failures or recurrent miscarriages.

According to Saxena, Mishra and Malik (2012), there are two types of surrogacy – traditional and gestational. In traditional surrogacy, the surrogate mother is impregnated with semen from the intended father. The surrogate is genetically related to the child, as her own eggs are used. She can conceive either by sexual intercourse or by an insemination procedure conducted at home/clinic. Traditional surrogacy, due to its legal concerns and consequences, is not permitted in most countries. In gestational surrogacy, the surrogate acts only as a 'carrier' of the embryo, which is not related to her genetically, as her own eggs have not been used. Pregnancy is conceived by IVF and the embryo is transferred into the womb (uterus) of the surrogate. The embryo can be the result of fertilization of gametes of the commissioning parents, or may be as a result of anonymous gamete donor fertilized with the gamete from one of the intended parents.

Both traditional and gestational surrogacy may be further classified as commercial and altruistic surrogacy. In commercial surrogacy, the surrogate is given monetary compensation to carry the child. This procedure is legalized in India. Many terms have been used for this type of pregnancy, like 'womb for rent', 'outsourced pregnancy', and 'baby farming'. In altruistic surrogacy, the surrogate does not gain any financial benefit for carrying the baby, but is compensated for her time. Her pregnancy-related expenditure is borne by the intended parents, such as medical and maternity expenses, travel to the IVF clinic, better quality food, etc. It is very difficult to source altruistic surrogates in today's times.

Surrogacy in modern times

The modern concept of surrogacy dates back to the mid-1970s, when the first 'official' legal surrogacy agreement was enacted in the USA by the lawyer Noel Keane (Utian et al., 1985). The birth of Louise Joy Brown, the world's first 'test-tube' baby, in 1978 paved the way for what is today known as gestational surrogacy. There was a great deal of controversy following the birth of 'Baby M' in 1985 in a partial surrogacy arrangement, and legislation (Surrogacy Arrangements Act, 1985) was rapidly passed to curb its practice. Under this law, commercial surrogacy arrangements were made illegal. After a great deal of discussion, in 1990 the British Medical Association finally agreed and set out guidelines for doctors intending to treat patients by gestational surrogacy – mainly suggesting that it should only be carried out for exceptional reasons after intensive investigation and counseling. The Human Fertilization and Embryology Act was passed in the year 1990 in the UK, and surrogacy was legalized.

In recent times, surrogacy has gone on to scale new heights of popularity. In fact, in 2005, a 58-year-old woman donned the role of surrogate mother to give birth to her own twin granddaughters. Since time immemorial, surrogacy has acted as a ray of hope for people who are unable to take the conventional route to parenthood. In addition, it may also be a survival strategy for those underprivileged women who carry a baby to earn a buck.

Surrogacy in India

India legalized gestational surrogacy in the year 2002, though traditional surrogacy is not legal. The exact prevalence of surrogacy in India is difficult to estimate, but India has become the preferred destination for reproductive tourism. According to Nigam and Ahmad (2013), the main reasons for this preference are the relatively low costs (50% less than surrogacy packages in other countries), efficient medical professionals who speak English, excellent infrastructure and facilities with ART clinics in each city, easy availability of commercial surrogates and availability of legal surrogacy services even for single men.

A study by the Confederation of Indian Industry in 2012 estimated that nearly 10,000 foreign couples visit India yearly for reproductive services and 30% of them are either single or homosexual. They have estimated that this industry generates an income of around 2.3 million US dollars annually.

A booming IVF industry, with no pre-existing guidelines, legislation or any regulatory body, paved the path for the conception of India's 'National Guidelines for Accreditation, Supervision & Regulation of ART Clinics' in 2002 (Sharma et al., 2002). The draft of this document was subjected to a huge public debate, with various suggestions received from the National Commission for Women and the National Human Rights Commission. These guidelines were finalized and published in 2005 (Sharma et al., 2005).

On obtaining feedback from different states of the country, it was noted that these guidelines were not being adhered to, and many unethical practices prevailed. Hence, the Indian Council of Medical Research (ICMR) developed its ART bill in 2008, which was again subjected to extensive public debate at national and international levels. Based on the comments received from various sources, the draft bill was revised and finalized in 2010 (Sharma and Bhargawa 2010).

According to the finalized version of the draft bill, a surrogate should be 21 to 35 years of age and should not have had more than five successful live births in her life, including her own children. The surrogate should be medically examined and tested for sexually transmitted and communicable diseases, which could be hazardous for the baby. She is also expected to declare in writing that she has not been the recipient of blood or blood products in the past six months. Anyone can act as a surrogate in India – known or unknown, related or unrelated. However, in the case of a relative acting as a surrogate, she should belong to the same generation as the commissioning mother. With regards to embryo transfer, the bill prohibits simultaneous embryo transfer in the intended mother. A surrogate is allowed to undergo embryo transfer a maximum of three times for the same couple. The bill is still in a draft stage at the time of writing, and needs to be passed in the Indian Parliament before it becomes a law.

The draft ART bill further proposes stringent guidelines for foreigners and nonresident Indian couples opting for surrogacy in India. The draft bill seeks to monitor the unregulated ART sector. The guidelines are:

- A tourist visa is not the appropriate visa category, and such foreigners will be liable to action for violation of visa conditions. The appropriate visa category for commissioning surrogacy is a medical visa.
- Foreign men and women intending to commission surrogacy should be duly married and the marriage should be sustained for at least two years prior to surrogacy. Current Indian laws do not recognize gay marriages.
- The couple commissioning surrogacy should be in possession of a letter from their country's embassy in India, or from the Foreign Ministry of their country, stating clearly that a) the country recognizes surrogacy; and b) the child/children to be born to the commissioning couple through the Indian surrogate will be permitted entry into their country as a biological child/ children of the commissioning surrogacy.
- The couple commissioning surrogacy is required to furnish an undertaking that they would take care of the child/children born through surrogacy.
- The couple should produce a duly notarized agreement between the applicant and the prospective Indian surrogate mother.
- The treatment concerning surrogacy should be done only at one of the registered ART clinics recognized by ICMR.
- Foreign couples, before leaving India for their return journey, require exit permission and should be carrying a certificate from the ART clinic confirming that the custody of the child/children has been taken by the couple, and the liabilities towards the Indian surrogate mother have been fully discharged as per the agreement. A copy of the birth certificate(s) of the child/children is needed by the Foreigner Regional Registration Office (FRRO) along with photocopies of the passport and visa of the commissioning parents.

These ICMR guidelines are voluntarily followed by ART clinics, which, in turn, are registered with ICMR for ART. Only clinics which fulfill ICMR's criteria are registered as accredited clinics and recommended to practice surrogacy. Countries like the USA issue medical visas for surrogacy only if the ART clinic is registered with ICMR. Since the ART bill is not a law as of now, clinics not following these guidelines are not punishable by law. However, the ART Regulation draft bill of 2010 has now become a part of the Cabinet Notes. It is expected that legislation regarding surrogacy in India will become stronger after this bill is passed, thus ensuring fairer and regulated practices.

The legal process

Legally, the surrogate agrees to forfeit her privacy and not to place the baby at risk by any 'high-risk behavior' such as taking nonprescription drugs, smoking or alcohol consumption. Her husband has to submit himself to a medical examination and abstain from practicing sex at certain times, as deemed appropriate by the doctor, which may be told to them time and again and can never be ensured unless the surrogate is put in a surrogate home for the entire nine months of pregnancy. Restricting the surrogate to the four walls of a dormitory or some nursing home in this way separates the surrogate from her children and husband.

Globally, in whichever country surrogacy is allowed, including India, the primary condition is that at least one of the intended parents should be biologically related. Thus a scenario where either of the intended parents is not biologically related is not permitted. In India, traditional surrogacy is not legal. As per the draft ART bill of 2010, the third-party donor and the surrogate mother have to relinquish all parental rights concerning the offspring in writing. Having said that, we can never completely curb the emotions of the mother that carries the baby.

All parties must agree to provide affidavits, a court appearance and testimony to effectuate the designated mother and father of the unborn baby. The courts honor contracts and agreements between the surrogate and the commissioning parents, unless circumstances significantly change, jeopardizing the best interests of the child. The surrogate mother is required to register as a patient in her own name, but the intended parents are considered as the legal parents of the baby, and the birth certificate contains the names of the intended parents.

Surrogacy organization

India has become the globally preferred surrogacy destination due to excellent standards of medical care and easy availability of surrogates, both at affordable prices. Desperate childless couples embark on the journey of parenthood through a surrogate's help.

The process starts with in-depth consultation and counseling of the intended parents and the surrogate on all aspects, including medical, legal, ethical and social. The intended parents undergo a complete medical examination, screening for infectious and communicable diseases, along with semen analysis of the male and ovarian reserve testing of the female partner. The surrogate also undergoes a complete medical checkup, screening for infectious diseases and testing of her womb, along with legal and psychological counseling.

Counseling includes advice on nutrition and abstinence, the possibility of pregnancy risks, multiple pregnancies, the need for hospitalization, cesarean deliveries, financial gains and the possible sense of bereavement on giving away the baby. A local guardian or caretaker is appointed to take care of the surrogate through the pregnancy. The caretaker's expenses are to be borne by the intended parents, though many times they take a small chunk from the surrogate as well.

The involved parties (intended parents along with the surrogate and her husband/close relative) sign a surrogacy agreement, which is a legal document. The intended parents and surrogate also sign some agreements with the clinic where the treatment is going to be carried out. The surrogate's spouse, or a close relative if she is widowed or divorced, is an involved party and needs to be in full agreement to her undergoing surrogacy.

The surrogates are admitted to surrogate homes after the embryo transfer for the first three and last two to three months of pregnancy, as these are the crucial months. However, her family is allowed to visit her. The first three months are crucial because there is a higher risk of miscarriage in these months. The last two months of pregnancy are critical as there is a risk of going into pre-term labor. Many a time, we have experienced that staying away from her family takes a toll on the surrogate and she makes excuses such as her child being unwell, or loss of a parent, in order to be allowed to go home earlier.

On the other hand, if the surrogate is divorced or separated, bearing in mind the social stigma and the secrecy involved, she prefers to stay in the dormitory/ surrogate home for the entire pregnancy. Rudrappa (2012), in her field study on surrogates in a surrogate home in the Indian city of Bangalore, found that the surrogates are well taken care of in these homes, and eventually they befriend the other surrogates staying there. In a way, they also get some time off from the burden of working round the clock for their families. While in the surrogate home, they follow a disciplined timetable, and a better balanced diet suiting their needs. Husbands are allowed to visit but cannot stay overnight. This is to make sure that no sexual relations take place.

Some surrogate homes have leisure activities as well: surrogates are taught English and to use computers. This may be done so that they can effectively communicate with the intended parents and keep them in the loop of day-to-day happenings, which is critical in such long-distance pregnancies.

Pande (2010), in her research on surrogacy, found that needy women are identified, persuaded and recruited into surrogacy. These are the women with economic desperation. For most of these surrogates, the money earned through surrogacy is equivalent to five years of total family income.

The problems faced by the intended parents are long-distance pregnancy: the language barrier; multiple trips to India, first to get themselves registered, then to deposit their gametes and finally to take away their child; a long stay away from home to complete the legal formalities and issues like DNA tests not matching, the nationality of the child, etc. Although daily communication from their doctors overcomes the geographical distance to a great extent, the parents still tend to be worried. Pregnancy check-ups, sonography images and videos are shared on a regular basis to help the intended parents stay at peace.

Surrogacy: the good, the bad and the ugly

Surrogacy is a complex and challenging subject that has been plagued with controversies for the past several decades. Surrogacy is a good option for selected couples, where genetic offspring is possible with good pregnancy rates, but the unhealthy combination of profit-driven clinics and financially desperate surrogates has led to many unethical practices in India. This has been observed by Shetty in her study on India's unregulated surrogacy (2010).

At one end of the spectrum is the pain of infertility and craving for parenthood, and at the other end is the commercialization of the reproductive capacity of women. If carried out ethically, it is the biggest boon to infertile women who have a problem with their uteri in order to have their own biological children, and a blessing for the surrogates who need those financial resources for better education of their own children. Earning an amount through surrogacy for which they would otherwise have to toil hard for years gives surrogates a better quality of life by providing for their family, buying a place to live and sometimes providing better education for their children. Despite this, many have compared and contrasted surrogacy with sex work. It is hard to tell whether surrogates are exercising their own free will or are being coerced and exploited to fulfill material and financial needs by their husbands and in-laws. Women, as second-class citizens in the third world, are extremely vulnerable to commercialization and exploitation.

Undoubtedly, there is also the possibility that surrogacy may be inappropriately used as a convenience for nonmedical reasons, and at times has been equated to a form of dehumanizing labor and 'organ trafficking'. Women are forced by economic necessity to rent their wombs to so-called privileged ones, as observed by van Zyl and van Niekerk (2000) and Ber (2000). Quoting the legal experts, Anu et al. (2013) have stated in their study that 'If surrogacy becomes an avenue by which women in richer countries choose poorer women in our country to bear their babies, then it is economical exploitation, a kind of biological colonization'.

A study on the surrogacy industry by the NGO Centre for Social Research (CSR, 2013), *Surrogacy motherhood: ethical or commercial?*, supported by the Ministry Of Women and Child Development, showed that there is no payment structure for the surrogates. Around 46% of the respondents in Delhi, and 44% in Mumbai, said they received between Rs 3 lakh and Rs 3.99 lakh for being a surrogate mother. Among those interviewed, 68% in Delhi and 78% in Mumbai said they were employed mostly as domestic help earning more than Rs 3,000 lakh a month. The report also found that some ART clinics are using two surrogates simultaneously to increase the chances of getting a baby. They also observed that the expanding surrogacy system is negatively affecting the adoption of orphaned and destitute children.

The payment may differ from surrogate to surrogate in many ART centers. Pande (2010) observed that in the absence of any binding law or contract, intended parents have considerable freedom in deciding the amount and form of remuneration. Women recruited for surrogacy are illiterate or semi-literate. These women are not given any copy of the written contract; they are not even aware of the clauses contained therein. Most of them do not understand English, the language in which the contract is written.

According to Dhawan (2013), most surrogates have minimal understanding of the medical procedures they are subjected to, and in the case of a miscarriage, they receive only a fraction of the money. According to Kimbrell (1998), surrogate mothers are unaware of their legal rights, and due to their financial status, cannot afford the services of lawyers, creating the possibility of exploitation.

On the other hand, there are centers which are ethical, counsel the surrogate along with her husband, explain the process, benefits and risks, explain the clauses of the contract and have the compensation included in the surrogate's contract, so that the intended parents and the surrogate both know exactly how much is being paid to the surrogate. They also make sure that the caretaker is paid by the intended parents, and not by the surrogate.

According to Ombelet et al. (2005) and Hansen et al. (2009), malpractices, such as transferring more than three embryos at a time, have resulted in multiple pregnancies, leading to increased maternal and neonatal morbidity and mortality, as well as excess economic burden.

In a retrospective study of 300 surrogates by Shah and Soni (unpublished data) at Hiranandani Hospital, Mumbai, 58% had single pregnancies whereas 42% had twin pregnancies; 17% delivered vaginally and 83% delivered by cesarean section. Pre-term delivery occurred in 18.7%, premature rupture of membranes in 30%, and 19.39% of infants had neonatal intensive care unit admissions. High blood pressure developed in 13.6% of surrogates, anemia in 6.9%; 17.5% had bleeding during pregnancy.

The issue of concern to the commissioning couples is that the surrogate may wish to retain the custody of the child due to emotional problems after having to relinquish the child. Studying the emotions of surrogates, a study by Jadva (2003) has shown that the majority of the surrogates do not experience psychological problems whilst handing over the baby, because they have their own children and do not crave another child, which would be an additional and unaffordable financial burden for them. They do have some emotional problems due to the reactions around them, which decrease within a few weeks following birth (Singh 2008). Regardless of their emotions for having given away a baby that their womb nurtured, Rudrappa (2012) found that the surrogates derive pleasure from securing their family's future and helping an infertile couple extend their family.

Another concern is the infringement of a newborn's fundamental right to its mother's milk. According to Jacobsson (2004), commissioning mothers find difficulty in initiating breast feeding and in establishing a bond between mother and child, resulting in the need for lactation being induced. According to Van den Akker (2007) and Golombok et al. (2013), one of the major drawbacks of induced lactation is that mothers rarely produce the same quantity of breast milk as a new mother immediately following childbirth. This poses a problem in terms of infant nutrition.

Golombok et al. (2013) did a longitudinal study to assess the psychological adjustment of children born through reproductive donation. The study concluded that children born through third-party reproduction had normal SDQ (Strengths and Difficulties Questionnaire) scores. Children born through surrogacy showed higher levels of adjustment at seven years of age versus children born through gamete donation. Children who were aware of the circumstances of their birth were more vulnerable to the effects of maternal distress. The lack of a gestational connection placed the children at increased psychological risk.

Conclusion

Surrogacy may be a simultaneous boon and a bane, just as any great technology or discovery. Gestational surrogacy, alternately hailed and criticized by one and all, is an excellent means to assist those desperate couples who cannot bear a child. However, the commercial and contractual nature of this arrangement still haunts its opponents.

Gestational surrogacy should be a part of comprehensive infertility treatment programs in accredited centers, with a full backup of lawyers, counselors and ethics committees. The government should seriously consider enacting a law to regulate surrogacy in India in order to protect the intended parents, the surrogate, the child born through surrogacy and the ART centers, thus preventing exploitation of any of them. The proposed law needs proper discussion and debate on legal, social, ethical and medical aspects. The main areas to be considered include the indications for surrogacy, complete evaluation of the surrogate, full compensation, legal surrogacy agreements, establishing genetic relationship, readiness to manage unexpected mishaps to the surrogate mother or child, ensuring the child's custody and having a system of jurisdiction for disputes arising out of the agreement.

References

American Society of Reproductive Medicine (ASRM). 2012. *Surrogacy guidelines update, April, 2012.*

Anu, Pawan Kumar, Deep Inder, Nandini Sharma. 2013. Surrogacy and women's right to health in India: Issues and perspective. *Indian journal of Public Health* 57(2):65–70.

Ber, Rosalie. 2000. Ethical issues in gestational surrogacy. *Theor Med Bioeth* 21:153–69.

Brinsden, Peter R. 2003. Gestational surrogacy. *Human Reproduction Update* 9(5):483–491.

British Medical Association (BMA). 1996. Surrogacy: Ethical Considerations. Report of the working Party on Human Infertility Services. London: BMA Publications.

Centre for Social Research (CSR). 2013. *Surrogate Motherhood – Ethical or Commercial.* February 2013, Surrogacy online report. Retrieved from http://www.womenleadership. in/Csr/SurrogacyReport.pdf.

Dhawan, H. 2013. Unregulated surrogacy industry worth over $2bn thrives without legal framework. *The Times of India*, July 18.

Golombok, Susan, Lucy Blake, Polly Casey, Gabriela Roman, Vasanti Jadva. 2013. Children Born Through Reproductive Donation: A Longitudinal Study of Psychological Adjustment. *J Child Psychol Psychiatry* 54(6):653–660.

Hansen, Michele, Lyn Colvin, Beverly Petterson, Jennifer Kurinczuk, Nicholas de Clerk, Carol Bower. 2009. Twins born following assisted reproductive technology: perinatal outcome and admission to hospital. *Human Reproduction* 24(9):2,321–2,331.

Jacobsson, Bo, Lars Ladfors, Ian Milsom. 2004. Advanced maternal age and adverse perinatal outcome. *Obstetrics and Gynecolgy* 104:727–733.

Jadva, Vasanti, Clare Murray, Emma Lycett, Fiona MacCullum, Susan Golombok. 2003. Surrogacy: the experiences of surrogate mothers. *Human Reproduction* 18:2,196–2,204.

Kimbrell, Andrew. 1998. *The Human Body Shop: The Cloning, Engineering, and Marketing of Life.* Washington DC: Regnery Publishing Inc.

Nigam, Aruna and Ayesha Ahmad. 2013. Surrogacy – An Indian perspective. *Tropical Clinics of Obstetrics and Gynaecolgy*, October 7.

Ombelet, W., Petra De Setter, Josiane Van der Elst, Guy Martens. 2005. Multiple gestation and infertility treatment. *Human Reproduction Update* 11(1):3–14.

Pande, Amrita. 2010. Commercial surrogacy in India: Manufacturing a perfect mother-worker. *Signs: Journal of Women in Culture and Society* 35(4):969–992.

Rudrappa, Sharmila. 2012. Indian reproductive assembly line. *Contexts* 11(2):23–27.

Saxena, Pikee, Archana Mishra, Sonia Malik. 2012. Surrogacy: ethical and legal issues. *Indian J Community Med* 37:211–13.

Shah, Duru and Anita Soni. Unpublished data.

Sharma, R.S., P.M. Bhargava, N. Chandhiok and N.C. Saxena. 2005. National guidelines for accreditation, supervision & regulation of ART clinics in India. New Delhi: Indian Council of Medical Research-Ministry of Health & Family Welfare, Government of India.

Sharma, R.S., P.M. Bhargava, N. Chandhiok and N.C. Saxena. 2002. New Delhi: Draft National guidelines for accreditation, supervision & regulation of ART clinics in India. Indian Council of Medical Research.

Sharma, R.S. and P.M. Bhargava. 2010. Draft, The Assisted Reproductive Technologies (Regulation) Bill. New Delhi: Ministry of Health and Family Welfare, Government of India; Indian Council of Medical Research.

Shetty, Priya. 2010. India's unregulated surrogacy industry. *The Lancet* 380(9854):1,633–1,634.

Singh, K.K. 2008. Human genome and human rights: An overview. *J Indian Law Inst* 50:67–80.

Surrogacy Arrangements Act. 1985. London: Her Majesty's Stationary Office.

Utian, Wilf, L. Sheean and J.M. Godfarb. 1985. Successful pregnancy after IVF and embryo transfer from an infertile women to a surrogate. *N England Journal Medicine* 313:1,351–1,352.

Van den Akker, Ola B. 2007. Psychological traits and state characteristics, social support and attitudes to the surrogate pregnancy and baby. *Human Reproduction* 22:2,287–2,295.

van Niekerk, Anton and Liezl van Zyl. 1995. The ethics of surrogacy: women's reproductive labour. *Journal of medical ethics* 21:345–349.

van Zyl, Liezl and Anton van Niekerk. 2000. Interpretations, perspectives and intentions in surrogate motherhood. *J Med Ethics* 26:404–409.

9 Circumvention, crisis and confusion

Australians crossing borders to Thailand for international surrogacy[1]

Andrea Whittaker

Introduction

The spread of ARTs throughout the world, combined with the ease of international travel and local restrictions, has produced a growing trade involving Australians travelling for international commercial surrogacy. Surrogacy may be used to enable couples who are unable to gestate a pregnancy due to medical reasons, such as the absence of a uterus in a woman, inability to carry a pregnancy, cases of recurrent failed implantation, recurrent idiopathic miscarriage or when a single male or same-sex male couple use ARTs to have children. Travelling for surrogacy services has been described as a form of 'circumvention travel', i.e. travel to receive medical services that are banned or restricted elsewhere or unavailable for those whose status makes them ineligible for treatments (as is the case with many treatments for infertility due to age, marital status or sexual orientation). These include certain states of the US, Ukraine, India and, until recently, Thailand. Those travelling for reproductive services sometimes self-describe as 'reproductive exiles', drawing attention to what they consider to be the 'forced' nature of their travel (Inhorn and Patrizio, 2009).

There are various forms of surrogacy. The term 'traditional' surrogacy is used to describe arrangements whereby a surrogate supplies her ova, gestates and gives birth to a child who is then handed over to be raised by another person or couple, known as the 'intending parent(s)' (a term used more frequently in Australia than *intended parents*). 'Gestational' surrogacy is the more common form of surrogacy, in which the surrogate has no biological relationship to the child produced. In gestational surrogacy the oocytes and/or sperm used to create the embryo(s) through in vitro fertilisation (IVF) can be either from the intending parents or from a donor or donors. The embryo is transferred to the gestational surrogate, who carries the pregnancy and gives birth to the child, who is then handed over to the intending parents.

In this chapter I analyse the experiences of Australians travelling to Thailand for surrogacy, citing cases that highlight the legal complexities involved in international cross-border surrogacy arrangements. In this chapter, I draw upon media reports, interviews with intending parents in Thailand and Australia, secondary material such as public Facebook discussions and key informant interviews with Thai medical officials, and argue that the booming global trade in surrogacy has created a number of legal and social challenges, particularly when surrogacy arrangements involve parties in different countries across jurisdictional borders. International surrogacy arrangements may conflict with home country regulations and legislation, exposing couples to potential legal consequences and resulting in difficulties in the establishment or recognition of the legal parentage of children. This may affect the child's nationality, immigration status and the attribution of parental responsibility regarding the child. All parties involved in such international arrangements are vulnerable. By acting beyond their state's jurisdiction, citizens remove themselves from their state's regulatory reach and protections, leaving them few legal protections or rights in either jurisdiction.

The first part of this chapter provides an overview of surrogacy and the demand for surrogacy services by Australians. The second part describes the legal context of surrogacy in Australia and Thailand. The use of surrogacy is highly controversial in many countries due to a range of ethical, religious and legal concerns, and as a result many countries ban or greatly restrict the forms and conditions under which surrogacy can take place. Jurisdictions that allow commercial surrogacy have liberal regulatory regimes, or little or no regulation, and include certain states of the United States of America, Ukraine and India. Thailand was an Asia-Pacific hub for surrogacy until recent changes in its regulatory environment made it difficult for potential parents and surrogates to transact, highlighting the potential for boundaries of surrogacy to change, and thus increasing the vulnerabilities of intending parents and surrogates. The third part of this chapter explores how these legal boundaries became critical to a set of cases involving children born through surrogacy arrangements in Thailand for Australian intending parents.

Australian surrogacy laws: incentives to seek assistance overseas?

The number of Australian parents having children through regulated surrogacy arrangements within Australia annually is very low ($n = 14$ in 2010). In contrast, according to a 2011 self-report survey of 14 surrogacy agencies in India, the US and Thailand, over 270 babies were born to Australians through overseas arrangements in the same period (Everingham et al., 2014; Macaldowie et al., 2013). The reasons people travel overseas for surrogacy is partly due to the difficulties in arranging surrogacy in Australia, the complex legal mosaic across the different states of Australia, the difficulties in locating a potential surrogate and perceived emotional complexity. As Millbank (2012) notes, within the last 25 years in Australia, surrogacy laws have been liberalised considerably, and altruistic surrogacy accepted as an unusual but legitimate means of family formation for the infertile; yet it remains legally complex and difficult. Under Australia's federal system, laws pertaining to surrogacy in Australia vary from state to state (see Table 9.1) and reflect the outcome of differing political concerns, histories of legislation and parliamentary debates. Surrogacy is highly regulated, aiming to protect all parties involved to prevent the possible exploitation of

Table 9.1 Legislation relating to surrogacy in all states and territories of Australia

Legislation relating to surrogacy		Traditional surrogacy allowed	Gestational altruistic surrogacy allowed	Ban on O/S commercial surrogacy
Australia	No Commonwealth legislation			
Australian Capital Territory	Parentage Act 2004	No	Yes	Yes, since 2004
New South Wales	Surrogacy Act 2010 No 102	Yes	Yes	Yes, since March 2011
Northern Territory	No legislation	Yes	Yes	No
Queensland	Surrogacy Act 2010	Yes	Yes	Yes, since 1988
South Australia	Statutes Amendment (Surrogacy) Act 2009	No	Yes	No
Tasmania	Surrogacy Act 2012	Yes	Yes	No
Victoria	Assisted Reproductive Treatment Act 2008 (Part 4, Surrogacy)	Not via a registered ART provider	Yes	No
Western Australia	Surrogacy Act 2008, Family Court (Surrogacy) Rules 2009 & Surrogacy Regulations 2009	No	Yes	No

Source: VARTA, www.varta.org.au/regulation/legislation-and-guideline-overview; Surrogacy Australia (n.d.)

women who act as birth mothers and protect the interests of children born through these means (Millbank, 2011).The only forms of surrogacy legal in states of Australia are those involving uncompensated or altruistic surrogacy, when the surrogate mother receives reimbursement only for out-of-pocket expenses (e.g. medical costs) associated with the pregnancy and birth. No commercial arrangements are permitted. Under these laws, altruistic surrogacy arrangements are not enforceable, i.e. a surrogate mother cannot be compelled to hand over a child after birth to the intending parents. States vary in the definitions of who is eligible to act as a surrogate, the level of counselling required, legal costs, what costs may be reimbursed and whether a regulatory authority is involved. In all states it is illegal to advertise for a surrogate, or for a surrogate to advertise.

For those couples who do undertake altruistic surrogacy arrangements in Australia, the current policy forbids the public universal health insurance scheme, Medicare, from providing rebates for IVF use for surrogacy. This is a further disincentive against couples pursuing surrogacy within Australia, as on average couples wanting to do an IVF cycle for surrogacy purposes are forced to pay AUD 12,000–18,000 (USD 8,325–12,488) compared to usual out-of-pocket expenses of around AUD 1,500 (USD 1,040) for couples covered by Medicare (Surrogacy Australia, n.d.).

Australians travelling overseas for surrogacy

It is unclear exactly how many Australians are travelling for surrogacy overseas. A retrospective audit of overseas surrogacy agencies carried out in 2011 by a parent support association, Surrogacy Australia, showed a 277% increase in the number of infants born to Australians via surrogacy, with numbers rising from 97 in 2009 to 269 in 2011 (Everingham et al., 2014; Everingham, 2014). Although not a random representative sample, an online survey of 1,135 members of two support groups, Gay Dads Australia and Surrogacy Australia, yielded 259 respondents who were considering surrogacy, were currently undertaking an uncompensated or compensated/commercial surrogacy agreement or had done so in the past. Mean total estimated costs of successful surrogacy were higher for the United States (AUD 172,347) compared with India (AUD 69,212). Among those who already had one or more children through surrogacy, 40% (41/103) described themselves as likely, very likely or definitely going to undertake surrogacy again in the future.

The destinations for commercial surrogacy reflect changes in regulatory regimes as well as cost and accessibility. Among Australians, the US states of California and New Jersey were the primary destinations for commercial surrogacy prior to 2009. India then became popular until 2012, when new visa regulations restricted access to married heterosexual couples. Since 2011, Thailand has grown in popularity as a destination (Everingham et al., 2014). As will be described in this chapter, since 2015, a change in legislation in Thailand restricted the availability of commercial surrogacy there. However, the international demand for surrogacy is strong, and in the wake of restrictions in one country, the endlessly flexible capitalist market ensures another destination will appear.

There is little information available on the outcomes for Australian couples of international surrogacy arrangements. However, results from a survey conducted in 2014 suggest that overseas surrogacy arrangements for Australians have had poor outcomes due largely to the practice of multiple embryo transfer in foreign clinics resulting in high-risk pregnancies. The survey of 259 members of two surrogacy support organisations (Stafford-Bell, Everingham & Hammarberg, 2014) found a high proportion (55%, 62/112) reported that their overseas surrogate had experienced multiple pregnancies due to the transfers of multiple embryos and there was a high rate (45%, 35/78) of premature birth. Ten per cent of those respondents surveyed (11/112) reported that a pregnancy had ended in a late miscarriage or perinatal death.

There is little qualitative research about Australians travelling overseas for surrogacy. A thesis (Stockey-Bridge, 2015) documents the travel of Australians to undertake commercial surrogacy arrangements in India. The Australian couples she followed described transnational surrogacy as their only hope of forming a family. Each couple had a different trajectory and experiences leading to the surrogacy clinics of India. Some resorted to surrogacy following traumatic reproductive histories and multiple attempts using IVF; some had unsuccessfully tried to adopt children but encountered bureaucratic difficulties in doing so and were either considered ineligible or were too old once the various hurdles had been overcome. Some gay couples had considered co-parenting arrangements as a means to biological fatherhood but preferred a surrogacy arrangement for its lack of complicated relationships. Many were deeply concerned about the ethics of their transactions and concerned about possible exploitation of overseas surrogates. In most cases they had little opportunity to meet or develop a relationship with their surrogate, and language differences usually limited their interactions.

In recognition that many couples seek surrogacy overseas, the Victorian Assisted Reproductive Treatment Authority (VARTA) prepared a 'Patient and physician prompter' and a 'Legal checklist' for parents considering surrogacy arrangements overseas. The legal checklist details a daunting range of legal issues that need to be considered, such as: questions covering the legal status of the arrangement in both countries and states; the conditions and rights of the surrogate; payments; problems within the pregnancy; legal status of the child and repatriation (http://www.varta.org.au/ivf-or-surrogacy-overseas/). It advises that couples need expert legal advice in both countries before undertaking any arrangement.

Australian citizenship for children born through overseas surrogacy

A child born overseas as a result of a surrogacy arrangement may be eligible for Australian citizenship by descent if at least one of the intended parents is an Australian citizen and the person with legal guardianship of the child consents to the application. The Australian Citizenship Act (2007) and Australian Citizenship Instructions set out the legal requirements for such applications. They require evidence that the child is the biological child of the intended parent(s), usually involving DNA testing and a certified copy of the surrogacy contract (despite the fact that such contracts are not enforceable under Australian law). As the existing legal guardian of the child, the surrogate mother is also required to consent to the application and may be interviewed by immigration staff at the Embassy (Australian Embassy Thailand, n.d.). This process ensures children are not left stateless and may obtain an Australian passport. However, it does not necessarily mean the child may leave the country, as this is dependent upon local laws in the country where the surrogacy birth has taken place.

Australian parentage versus parenting orders

A confusing legal maze confronts Australian parents of children born through overseas commercial surrogacy arrangements. Parentage laws ensure that children have a legal relationship with the parents who are raising them and also vary from state to state (see Table 9.2). At the moment, under Australian law there are different categories depending on where surrogacy takes place. Under Section 60H of the Family Law Act, within Australia a surrogate mother (and her consenting partner) are presumed to be the parents of the child. It is necessary for intending parents to obtain a 'parentage order', which is made in the Supreme Court, whereby the status of parent is conferred upon the intending parents, who may then apply for a new birth certificate with their names. The requirements for obtaining a parentage order also vary in each state and territory (Millbank, 2011).

Intending parents who have gone through a commercial arrangement overseas cannot apply for a parentage order available to those in altruistic arrangements under state and territory surrogacy legislation, regardless of genetic link, whether they are named on a foreign birth certificate or court order. This is because half of the Australian state legislative regimes exclude children conceived outside the jurisdiction, and all exclude arrangements where payment has been made to the

Table 9.2 Legislation relating to donor treatment procedures and parentage throughout Australia

Australia	Family Law Act 1975
Australian Capital Territory	Parentage Act 2004
New South Wales	Status of Children Act 1996
Northern Territory	Status of Children Act 1979
Queensland	Status of Children Act 1978
South Australia	Family Relationships Act 1975
Tasmania	Status of Children Act 1974
Victoria	Status of Children Act 1974; Human Tissue Act 1982
Western Australia	Artificial Conception Act 1985

Source: VARTA, www.varta.org.au/regulation/legislation-and-guideline-overview

birth mother (Millbank, 2011). Rather, the only recourse to them is to apply to the Family Court for a 'parenting order' conferring parental responsibility upon them. This does not make them the legal parents of the child, but it permits them to function as parents and exercise parental responsibility. As a result of the perceived legal complexity, legal costs and the fact that parenting orders are not required in most settings including for school enrolment or public medical insurance, many parents who have children born through international surrogacy arrangements never apply for parenting orders. This has implications for the children born through such arrangements; for example, in matters of inheritance, if they are not named in a will they may have no support or entitlement. There are also potential difficulties in cases of divorce or relationship breakdown.

In international surrogacy arrangements, foreign laws of parentage apply, leading to further complications and unpredictable outcomes for children born through surrogacy.

Extraterritorial laws: extending legal boundaries

Consistent with local bans on commercial or compensated surrogacy, three states (Queensland, New South Wales and the Australian Capital Territory) have enacted laws banning residents from facilitating or undertaking commercial surrogacy overseas. Legal cases, involving commercial surrogacy arrangements in Thailand, are revealing the human and ethical dilemmas involved in such a ban. The case of Dudley and Anor and Chedi (2011) in the Family Court of Australia [Fam CA 502 (30 June 2011)] involved a couple, residents of Queensland, who went to Thailand for overseas surrogacy. Both aged 42, the couple had tried IVF in Australia for ten years before seeking surrogacy overseas. They hired two surrogate mothers, one of whom had twin boys and the other one boy from donated eggs and the sperm of the father. The couple sought parental orders for the three boys in the Family Court in Sydney. In two separate cases by two judges, the parents were granted parental orders for the boys as it was judged in the children's best interests. However, one judge ordered the case to be referred to the Department of Public Prosecution in Queensland to consider whether the couple should be prosecuted for entering into a commercial surrogacy arrangement, which carries a three-year jail term.

Similarly, a second couple from Queensland who had undergone surrogacy in Thailand and sought parenting orders for the child (Findlay and Anor and Punyawong [2011] FamCA 503) was also referred to the Queensland Department of Public Prosecutions. In another case (Johnson and Anor and Chompunut [2011] FamCA 505), an Australian father seeking a parenting order for a child born in Thailand to an unwed Thai surrogate was denied status as a parent by the Australian Family Court because Thai authorities did not recognise the father of a child of an unwed Thai mother. They would be required to produce a court order relinquishing her rights as a parent, which under Thai law is not possible for an unwed mother until the child has reached seven or eight years of age. As a consequence, the child was not considered eligible for a visa on the basis of descent until such a court order had been produced. The judge involved also considered referring this case, and another (Hubert and Juntasa [2011] FamCA 504 (30 June 2011), for potential extraterritorial prosecution; but the relevant provisions were not yet in effect at the time the arrangements had been made.

These cases demonstrate the difficulties in enforcement and prosecution of extraterritorial laws and the legal quagmire that can result across different jurisdictions. Although these cases were not prosecuted, the families involved potentially faced jail terms of up to three years and fines for their actions in conducting a commercial surrogacy arrangement overseas, and the third family faced a period of legal limbo for their child. Unintended consequences of these laws may simply be to reinforce discrimination against certain groups of patients seeking to form families (such as infertile couples, or gay couples), force cross-border commercial surrogacy to go underground or be manipulated into appearing like altruistic surrogacy, make parents avoid seeking parental orders for their children depriving children of their legal status and potentially turn some parents into criminals.

These extraterritorial laws appear to have been ineffective as a deterrent to couples seeking surrogacy overseas. In the online survey of members of two surrogacy support groups (Everingham et al., 2014), 55% (63/113) of respondents from Australian states where the laws apply stated they would proceed with their plans to undertake overseas surrogacy regardless, given the low chance of prosecution, while 23% (26/113) stated they would move to a state where the laws did not apply. Millbank (2011) argues that the states' extraterritorial criminal sanctions and the categorical exclusion of children born through paid surrogacy from legal parentage regimes in Australian jurisdictions are insufficiently justified and ineffective. She suggests that 'criminalisation may inhibit constructive discussion about how domestic surrogacy could be expanded or international surrogacy made safer'.

Crisis and confusion: Thai surrogacy laws

The vulnerabilities and potential legal consequences of international surrogacy became overt in a series of highly publicised incidents in Thailand from 2011 to 2014 that eventually resulted in the passing of legislation restricting surrogacy. Until 2015, surrogacy in Thailand was regulated by professional guidelines issued by the Thai Medical Council in 1997 and 2001 (Announcements 1/2540 and 21/2544), which limited surrogacy to married couples, banned commercial transactions and stated that a surrogate must be a biological relative of the married couple (Virutamasen et al., 2001). However, these guidelines had no legislative force and a number of clinics appear to have ignored them.

Similarly, parentage laws in Thailand were also not conducive to surrogacy arrangements, yet intended parents managed to circumvent them. Under section 1546 of the Thai Civil and Commercial Code, the woman who gives birth to a child is regarded as the legal mother of that child. When a child is born to an unwed woman, she alone is recognised as having the legal rights over that child. Under the same code, the father of a child who is not married to the mother at the time of birth has no parental rights over that child even if recorded on the birth certificate or able to prove his biological parentage. In effect, a child born through surrogacy would have to be legally adopted for the parentage of the intending parents to be recognised.

With unsupportive guidelines and unfavourable parentage laws, Thailand was not a popular destination for commercial surrogacy until 2012, when Indian restrictions to their surrogacy policies helped stimulate interest in Thailand as a surrogacy destination. In October 2012, the Indian government passed regulations restricting the categories of visa legally available to foreign intending parents. These required people travelling to India for a surrogacy arrangement to apply for a surrogacy visa. These are only available to couples who have been married for a minimum of two years. Single men and women and same-sex couples are thus no longer legally able to apply for surrogacy in India. Within four months of this change, clinics lobbied and had the restrictions overturned; however, a ruling at the end of 2013 criminalising 'homosexual acts' again made travel to India by gay couples legally risky. It remains to be seen whether the new Indian Assisted Reproductive Technologies Bill will allow single people to apply for surrogacy. In contrast, around this time Thai clinics began blatantly advertising the availability of surrogates and egg donors and 'gay-friendly' services. A number of new clinics and facilitation companies openly promoted surrogacy in Thailand.

The first incident to reveal the illicit side of Thai commercial surrogacy involved the trafficking of Vietnamese women to act as surrogates for a Taiwanese company based in Bangkok. On 28 February 2011, Thai police raided a house owned by company Baby 101, a 'eugenics surrogate' company with offices in Bangkok, Phnom Penh and Vietnam and registered with the Russian Federation in Vladivostok. Fourteen Vietnamese women were found to have been trafficked to Thailand to work as surrogates for Taiwanese couples, receiving USD 5,000 per surrogacy (AAT, 2011). On 22 June 2012, the Thai Primary Court found four Taiwanese defendants in the case guilty of human trafficking and they were sentenced to 5.3 years in jail (AAT, 2012). Eventually the 11 babies involved were sent to their eight biological families in Taiwan. This case highlighted the lack of oversight and monitoring by clinics, the commodification of surrogacy and the vulnerability of poor women in the region to the growing trade. Despite public outrage within the Thai press at the time, this case prompted no widespread investigation into the industry.

Further controversial cases in 2014 drew public attention to the flagrant breaches of the medical guidelines in Thailand. These included a highly publicised case of Israeli intending parents whose babies born through surrogacy arrangements were stranded in Thailand as the Israeli government refused to grant them citizenship (Murdoch and Snow, 2014). In August 2014 another story broke in the media of a Japanese man, Mitsutoki Shigeta, who reportedly fathered 16 babies to multiple surrogate mothers in Thailand and had fled the country with at least three of the babies. The clinic involved in his case, ALL-IVF (one very popular with Australian couples) was closed pending investigation (Gecker and Doksone, 2014).

Baby Gammy

Of all the stories about surrogacy in Thailand in 2014, the story of Baby Gammy drew worldwide attention to the practice of international surrogacy across borders. In August 2014, the media ran the story of Baby Gammy, a baby boy with Down syndrome who had been abandoned in Thailand by his Australian intending parents (and biological father) to be cared for by his gestational surrogate (Whiteman, 2014; Murdoch, 2014). His twin sister had been taken back to Australia. The story broke after appeals from the surrogate, Ms Janbua Pattharamon, for support for Baby Gammy's medical expenses from international donors. She appeared in the media explaining that she had agreed to be a surrogate to pay off family debts and had refused an (illegal) abortion when it was discovered that one of the twins she was carrying had Down syndrome. Rather than institutionalise the boy child, she offered to care for him. The intending parents took the daughter and left the country, leaving the son with the surrogate mother (Murdoch, 2014). Following further media investigations it was revealed that the father in the case, Mr David Farnell, is a convicted sex offender who spent time in prison for sexually abusing young girls. Editorials called for the enforcement of bans against international surrogacy (Ekman, 2014; Mitchell, 2014; Wilson, 2014). The couple was placed under investigation by Australian authorities. Baby Gammy was granted Australian citizenship in January 2015 and remains in the care of his surrogate mother (Hawley, 2015).

The controversy in Australia continued when in August 2014 it was revealed in the media that another unnamed Australian man had been charged with the sexual abuse of his twin daughters conceived through surrogacy in Thailand. Subsequently, in the media it was claimed by a representative of the NGO Childline Thailand that the Thai government was considering repatriation of the girls to Thailand as an option, as the Thai surrogate remains the legal mother (Berkovic, 2014).

Reactions in Australia

Before these cases, reports of overseas surrogacy by Australians was attracting growing sympathy in the Australian media, with images of couples seeking surrogacy as vulnerable people being proactive in their attempts to form a family (Riggs and Due, 2013; 2014). The Baby Gammy case reversed this, and overseas surrogacy came to be depicted as an inherently dangerous, immoral and exploitative enterprise by opportunists with an overwhelming sense of privilege. For eager Australian intending parents, their dreams of forming a family through international surrogacy became heavily stigmatised (Murdoch and Snow, 2014). The perfect storm of an abandoned disabled child, a former sex offender father, a charismatic, caring and impoverished surrogate and an unscrupulous surrogacy agency all set within the context of a military coup and poorly regulated clinics caused embarrassment for the governments concerned as well as drawing worldwide attention to the difficulties of monitoring or regulating international cross-border transactions. There are calls for the need to review Australia's surrogacy compensation rules and bans on advertising for surrogates, to allow higher amounts of compensation to surrogates and make it easier for people to find women willing to act as surrogates (Millbank, 2014). The Chief Justice of the Family Court, Justice Diana Bryant, has called for a national review and the legalisation of commercial surrogacy in Australia to encourage couples to pursue surrogacy within Australia where careful regulation may ensure ethical arrangements and avoid abuses (Brennan, 2015).

Reactions in Thailand: new legislation

The avalanche of horrific media reports on practices surrounding commercial surrogacy in Thailand forced the government to act. On 22 July 2014, the military government, the National Peace and Order Council, announced a review of all 12 Thai IVF clinics involved in surrogacy cases believed to be possibly involved in breaches of the Thai Medical Council guidelines and not certified by the Royal College of Obstetricians. The next act of the NPOC was to revive the Assisted Reproductive Technologies Bill number 167/2553. Renamed 'The Protection of Children Born from Assisted Reproductive Technologies Act', it enforces a ban on commercial surrogacy or ova donation as well as non-medical sex selection and disallows intermediaries or brokers for surrogacy arrangements. The Act was published in the *Royal Gazette*, 1 May 2015, and took effect from 30 July 2015 (*Bangkok Post*, 2015). This new legislation strictly regulates the use of ARTs in Thailand and clarifies the legal status of children born through these technologies. Under the legislation, commercial surrogacy is not permitted (Section 23). It limits surrogacy to procedures using the ova and sperm of a Thai heterosexual married couple or using the ova or sperm of either a husband or wife paired with the sperm or egg of another donor. In the case of Thai citizens married to foreigners, they must have been married for a minimum of three years. A surrogate must be a Thai citizen and be biologically related to the couple. She must have had a child before, and if married, must have the permission of her husband before undergoing surrogacy. According to Wanlop Tankananurak, a member of Thailand's National Legislative Assembly, 'This law aims to stop Thai women's wombs from becoming the world's womb' (ABC News, 2015) through penalties including a maximum of ten years in jail and a fine of 200,000 baht (USD 5,538).

Section 25 of the legislation bans the facilitation of the trade by agents, brokers, clinics or facilitation companies and makes it an offence to accept financial or other benefits for the engagement or management of surrogacy. Section 26 also prohibits advertisements seeking women wishing to act as surrogates, whether for commercial purposes or otherwise.

Significantly, for Thai couples who will undertake surrogacy in the future, Section 27 of the draft surrogacy law removes the ambiguity over the parentage of a child born of surrogacy arrangements. It provides that a child born through means permitted under the ARTs Act will be deemed to be the legitimate child of the intending parents, not the surrogate or other person who provided genetic material.

Conclusions

A number of factors contributed to the development of Thailand as a site for the international surrogacy trade. These include push factors such as the heavily regulated and diverse state legislative frameworks in Australia for 'altruistic' surrogacy, which make it difficult, time consuming and uncertain. Similarly, adoption laws in Australia make adoption an extremely limited and time-consuming option. In addition, the growing movement for and social acceptance of gay biological fatherhood through surrogacy in Australia has created a new demand for surrogacy services. The growing wealth in recent years of Australians and the cheaper costs in countries such as India and Thailand made surrogacy affordable for more couples. The internet has allowed the proliferation of sites advertising surrogacy services, agencies and facilitators along with the growth of an internet community of parents through surrogacy normalising the practice.

On the Thai side, pre-existing expertise in assisted reproduction and a sophisticated medical tourist industry provided the infrastructure for the rapid growth of surrogacy services in private clinics. Laissez faire regulation through medical guidelines with no legislative framework provided little disincentive to clinics being involved in commercial surrogacy. Despite unfavourable parentage laws which only recognised the parentage of the birth mother, intending parents were able to negotiate Thai regulations to provide workable solutions allowing children to leave Thailand and be parented by Australian couples.

The series of cases highlighting the trafficking of women, the abandoning of disabled children, the poor regulation of the industry and the legal uncertainties for couples and their children shocked Thailand and Australia and revealed how borders not only separate and regulate, but potentiate and facilitate interactions. The trade in surrogacy thrives on differences. It is facilitated by marketable differences in jurisdiction, different enforcement of regulation, differences in economic status between surrogate mothers and intending parents and different ethical practices between clinics and doctors.

More broadly, the case of Thailand demonstrates how the international market in surrogates is in part attributable to and sustained by the domestic policies of source countries, many of which deem commercial surrogacy unethical. Travel across borders makes restrictive laws in Australia viable by exporting the proscribed activities. Current Australian domestic laws make it difficult to identify potential surrogates, and provide inadequate compensation for surrogates. The legislation banning overseas commercial surrogacy in three Australian states appears unworkable and difficult to enforce. The current mosaic of surrogacy legislation in Australia encourages Australians to travel overseas to pursue arrangements that are relatively quick, easily arranged, affordable and potentially anonymous.

Storrow (2005) has argued that countries have ethical obligations to take responsibility for the extraterritorial effects of their own reproductive policies. Some consider the need to reduce the number of infertile couples participating in the trade, hence reducing demand for the services of international surrogates (Parks, 2010). Millbank (2014) argues that domestic laws in Australia need reform to make it easier for Australian couples to find and undertake well-regulated domestic surrogacy arrangements. She proposes reform of current bans on advertising or facilitation of any form of surrogacy and restrictions on who can become a surrogate, which make it extremely difficult for couples to locate women willing to undertake altruistic arrangements if they do not have a pre-existing relationship. She suggests the introduction of a wage-based or risk-based compensation within Australia as well as public funding for ART, to remove incentives for couples to travel overseas. However, even if such changes were made to Australian surrogacy, it is likely that cost differences would still ensure the travel of some couples overseas.

Previously, I have detailed the difficulties in the various policy and legal approaches available to a state with regard to the regulation of cross-border medical trade including unilateral and multilateral options (Whittaker, 2010; Whittaker, 2011). Huge hurdles are faced to regulate ethical practices, provide consumer protections, restrict clinical procedures, regulate medical facilitators or harmonize legislative differences across jurisdictions if the harms revealed in the surrogacy industry in Thailand are to be avoided elsewhere (Whittaker, 2010: 406).

Note

1 Since this chapter was written the Thai government has passed the 'The Protection of Children Born from Assisted Reproductive Technologies Act', effective from 30 July 2015. The Act enforces a ban on commercial surrogacy and ova donation and restricts the eligibility for surrogacy to heterosexual couples (at least one of whom must be Thai) who must have been married for at least two years. Nepal also banned surrogacy on 25 August 2015.

References

ABC News. 2015. *Thailand bans surrogacy for foreigners in bid to end 'rent-a-womb' tourism*, 20 February 2015. Available: http://www.abc.net.au/news/2015-02-20/thailand-bans-surrogacy-for-foreigners/6163810

Alliance Anti Trafic (AAT). 2011. *The case of fifteen Vietnamese women recruited to become surrogate mothers in a baby-breeding ring in Thailand. Review of the international media coverage and the role of Alliance Anti-Trafic*, February/May 2011. Bangkok: Alliance Anti Trafic.

Alliance Anti Trafic (AAT). 2012. AAT Flash News. June 2012. [Accessed 9 August 2012.]

Australian Embassy Thailand. n.d. *Children born as a result of a surrogacy arrangement in Thailand* [Online]. Department of Immigration and Border Protection. Available: http://www.thailand.embassy.gov.au/bkok/DIAC_surrogacy_arrangement.html [Accessed 24 October 2014.]

Bangkok Post. 2015. *Law banning commercial surrogacy takes effect Thursday.* 29 July 2015. Available: http://www.bangkokpost.com/print/637960/ [Accessed 4 February 2016.]

Berkovic, N. 2014. Police checks urged in surrogacy cases. *The Australian*, Thursday, 4 September 2014.

Brennan, B. 2015. *Commercial surrogacy should be legalised, Family Court Chief Justice Diana Bryant says.* ABC News, 18 April 2015. Available: http://www.abc.net.au/news/2015-04-18/commercial-surrogacy-should-be-legalised-family-court-justice/6402924 [Accessed 4 February 2016.]

Ekman, K. E. 2014. Ban the baby trade before it grows any bigger. *Weekend Australian*, Saturday, 6 September 2014.

Everingham, S. 2014. Use of surrogacy by Australians: Implications for policy and law reform. *In:* Hayes, A. & Higgins, D. (eds), *Families, policy and the law: selected essays on contemporary issues for Australia.* Canberra: Australian Government, Australian Institute of Family Studies.

Everingham, S. G., Stafford-Bell, M. A. & Hammarberg, K. 2014. Australians' use of surrogacy. *The Medical Journal of Australia*, 201:270–273.

Gecker, J. & Doksone, T. 2014. Surrogate offers clues into man with 16 babies. *Associated Press: Worldstream*, Tuesday, 2 September 2014.

Hawley, S. 2015. *Baby Gammy, one-year-old at centre of Thai surrogacy scandal, granted Australian citizenship.* ABC News, 20 January 2015.

Inhorn, M. & Patrizio, P. 2009. Rethinking reproductive "tourism" as reproductive "exile". *Fertility and Sterility*, 92:904–906.

Macaldowie, A., Wang, Y. A., Chambers, G. M. & Sullivan, E. A. 2013. *Assisted reproductive technology in Australia and New Zealand 2010*, AIHW.

Millbank, J. 2011. New Surrogacy Parentage Laws in Australia: Cautious Regulation or 25 Brick Walls. *The. Melb. UL Rev.*, 35:165.

Millbank, J. 2012. From Alice and Evelyn to Isabella: Exploring the Narratives and Norms of New Surrogacy in Australia. *Griffith L. Rev.*, 21:101.

Millbank, J. 2014. Rethinking "Commercial" Surrogacy in Australia. *Journal of Bioethical Inquiry*, 1–14.

Mitchell, M. 2014. Time to strengthen our lax surrogacy laws – opinion: THEIR SAY. *Newcastle Herald (Australia)*.

Murdoch, L. 2014. Australian couple leaves Down syndrome baby with Thai surrogate. *The Age*, 1 August 2014.

Murdoch, L. & Snow, D. 2014. Rising distaste about paid pregnancy as Thai government moves to shut down industry. *The Age*, Saturday, 9 August 2014.

Parks, J. 2010. Care ethics and the global practice of commercial surrogacy. *Bioethics*, 24(7):333–340.

Riggs, D. W. & Due, C. 2013. Representations of reproductive citizenship and vulnerability in media reports of offshore surrogacy. *Citizenship studies*, 17:956–969.

Riggs, D. W. & Due, C. 2014. "The Contented Faces of a Unique Australian Family": Privilege and Vulnerability in News Media Reporting of Offshore Surrogacy Arrangements. *Feminist Media Studies*, 1–5.

Stafford-Bell, M. A., Everingham, S. & Hammarberg, K. 2014. Outcomes of surrogacy undertaken by Australians overseas. *The Medical Journal of Australia*, 201:330–333.

Stockey-Bridge, M. 2015. Finding Hope on the Transnational Surrogacy Trail from Australia to India. Unpublished PhD Thesis, Macquarie University, Sydney.

Storrow, R. F. 2005. Quests for Conception: Fertility Tourists, Globalization and Feminist Legal Theory. *Hastings Law Journal*, 57:295–330.

Surrogacy Australia. n.d. *Surrogacy and Medicare* [Online]. Available: http://www.surrogacyaustralia.org/ [Accessed 16 March 2015.]

Virutamasen, P., Pruksananonda, K., Limpaphayom, K., Chokevivat, V. & Kunaratanapruk, S. 2001. The regulation of assisted reproductive technology in Thailand. *Journal of the Medical Association of Thailand (Chotmaihet thangphaet)*, 84(10):1,490–1,494.

Whiteman, H. 2014. Surrogate mom vows to take care of ill twin 'abandoned' by parents. *CNN Wire*, Monday, 4 August 2014.

Whittaker, A. 2010. Challenges of medical travel to global regulation: A case study of reproductive travel in Asia. *Global Social Policy*, 10:287–291.

Whittaker, A. 2011. Cross-border assisted reproduction care in Asia: implications for access, equity and regulations. *Reproductive Health Matters*, 19:107–116.

Wilson, L. 2014. Surrogacy inquiry call. *The Advertiser (Adelaide, Australia)*.

10 Ethical aspects and legal problems when parents return home to Europe after cross-border surrogacy

Françoise Shenfield

Introduction

Ever since the beginnings of in vitro fertilization (IVF), national laws have responded to societal concerns about the status of and research on the embryo in vitro, and conditions of access to the many techniques of ARTs for women, whether married or not, in a couple or not, and (rarely) men in a same-sex relationship. Third-party reproduction involves the collaboration of people (sperm donors, egg donors, or surrogates) other than the "intended parents", also called "commissioning parents". From the onset, this complicates the professional responsibility which is already characterized in ART by the fact that this is engaged towards two patients, the intended parents, rather than one, like in most other fields of medicine. Furthermore, we also have to take into account the welfare of the future child, whether explicitly (HFE Act 1990, revised 2008)[1] or implicitly. In surrogacy arrangements, like in gamete donation, this also necessarily involves responsibility to third parties, and the usual bio-ethical frame of respecting the (infertile) patients' autonomous choice, optimizing their interests with maximizing beneficence and minimizing complications (non-maleficence), must be balanced with the essential respect of such donors/collaborators/third parties' interests and autonomy, more specifically avoiding their exploitation. Thus gamete donation has been one of the much discussed topics for many years (anonymous or known, compensated or even paid?), but whilst sperm donation is an "old" subject as it antedated the first IVF success by decades, only the latter technique enabled egg donation and full surrogacy, highlighting the specific female gender concerns when either is needed. However, amongst all issues of concern to society in the field, surrogacy,

> where a woman carries a pregnancy and delivers a child on behalf of a couple where the woman is unable to do so, because of a congenital or acquired uterine abnormality, or because of a serious medical contra indication to pregnancy, and where the intention is that the surrogate will relinquish the born child to the commissioning couple
>
> (FIGO ethics committee, 2008)

… has been one of the most contentious in ART, with concerns about the possible exploitation of women, and the instrumentalization of the female body. It is also possible for gay couples to use this technique to become parents, and this is legal in the UK and USA for instance, but the practice is probably more frequent in the latter. Surrogacy is illegal in many countries where ART is commonly practiced (such as France, Germany, Norway, or Spain), and sometimes "supported by specific legislation, enabling the commissioning couple to become the legal parents" (Greece, USA, UK), or even practiced if a specific law does not forbid it (Brunet et al., 2013).

Thus Europe, a leader in the field of ART, is far from homogeneous in its national law-making in ART and specifically concerning surrogacy, whilst the European Union (EU) has only officially intervened in two relevant fields: one practical, with the Tissue Directive which affects keeping gametes and embryos and their traceability (EU Tissue Directive, 2004), the other concerning the free movement of citizens across Europe in order to obtain treatment, therefore giving an official blessing to the phenomenon of cross-border reproductive care (CBRC) (EU Directive, 2011). CBRC may also involve further borders, between continents and/or between high and low resource areas in the world, highlighting other important issues, especially the possibility of exploitation of poor women by rich(er) women or couples.

In this chapter we discuss some of the legal issues which have made press titles and websites in Europe and worldwide (Sharp, 2014) and were recently detailed in several reports such as the one commissioned by the EU Directorate General for Internal Policies. Such legal problems vary, and involve either the lack of permission for commissioning couples to leave the birth country with their intended child(ren), or legal issues of parentage and nationality upon return to their home country, where surrogacy is (often) banned. They are also intrinsically linked to the ethical issues highlighted above, as ideally the ethical underpinning of justice should be clear. An important question is of course whether "justice" or the law in general is as ethical (just, equitable) as it purports to be semantically. As explained by Dickens (1997), emeritus Professor of Law in Toronto and past chairman of the International Federation of Gynaecology and Obstetrics Societies (FIGO)'s ethics committee, "law and ethics sometimes overlap and sometimes conflict". Thus, the purpose of this chapter is to give examples of both propositions, and to encourage means of achieving the "overlap" more often than the "conflict". To illustrate this, we will also discuss some of the jurisprudence of the European Court of Human Rights (ECt HR), a supranational European body whose renderings must be integrated in national law, and which may confirm or criticize national legislation on human rights grounds.

Before giving some examples of the legal issues which arose during the recent years when "intended" parents returned home after cross-border surrogacy, we first highlight specific ethical issues linked to CBRC and surrogacy, and use the example of the compensation for egg donors in order to reflect on the difficulties of defining fair compensation within a non-commercial system, as is practiced in Europe.

Specific ethical issues concerning CBRC and surrogacy

Infertile patients cross national borders in order to circumvent their home countries' restrictions on procedures, long waiting lists or legal constraints on eligibility, but the regulatory differences may also result in potential risks, especially difficulties for patients in pursuing any legal disputes in overseas jurisdictions, or difficulties upon their return home with a much wanted child. CBRC, a much preferred term to "tourism" as it does not penalize patients, is not wrong per se as it "enhances patients' autonomy, but safeguards must be observed, especially in case of third party ART" (ESHRE Ethics and Law Taskforce, 2009). The same ESHRE Task Force on Ethics and Law (2005) recommends in the case of surrogacy that "in order to ensure free and well-considered decision-making by the surrogate/gestating woman ... the woman has at least one child" and highlights single embryo transfer (ET) as best practice, as it diminishes complications for both the pregnant women and future babies it also states that the "gestational carrier's decisions during pregnancy [are] paramount". In its turn, FIGO's ethics committee recommended in 2008 that "In general, compensation for expenses directly related to the pregnancy, and loss of income due to the pregnancy, is accepted", stressing that "disproportionate payment given to surrogate women risks coercion of vulnerable women, and has the potential to lead to commercial exploitation, in particular recruitment of women of underprivileged background". Furthermore, surrogate arrangements should not be commercial, and are best arranged by non-profit agencies rather than brokers. Thus it highlights "trans-border reproductive agreements, where there is increased risk of coercion of resource poor women from resource rich countries". After the first international European study analyzing reasons for CBRC in six European countries (Shenfield et al., 2010), an ESHRE Taskforce on CBRC published a good practice guide to care for centers and practitioners (Shenfield, 2012) suggesting how to reduce risks and inequalities in CBRC, through abiding by the principles of equity, safety, efficiency, effectiveness, timeliness, and patient-centeredness. This guide also recommends single ET to the surrogates, as dangers of multiple pregnancies are well documented, due mainly to the complications of intrauterine growth retardation, preterm delivery, and their long term consequences for the children born, added to the risks for the pregnant woman. It is stressed that "single embryo transfer is the only acceptable option", and that "continuity of care during pregnancy and childbirth must be planned prior to starting the surrogacy cycle" (Shenfield et al., 2005; Shenfield et al., 2010). The guide further specifies that:

> the provision of legal advice about local rules is the remit of the local practitioner, or if not possible, through referral to appropriate local legal advisors, [and finally], in order to ensure free and well-considered decision-making by the surrogate/gestating woman, it is required that the surrogate candidate has at least one child.

Whilst safety must be paramount, the question of compensation for gamete donation or non-commercial surrogacy is also especially ethically sensitive, contrary to the contractual commercial basis in the USA, where payment for the "services" of the surrogate are mostly clearly set out prior to signature of the contract. The term "compensation" itself is prone sometimes to dogmatic interpretation, varying from the view that any payment is an affront to women's dignity, to an analysis of what amounts to a proportional and fair compensation. This may range from a refund of documented expenses only, to a lump sum covering expenses and time loss.

How to analyze this debated question of proportionate compensation more clearly may be illustrated here by a comparison with recent research performed with ESHRE colleagues on egg donors' characteristics and motivations in Europe (Pennings et al., 2014).

The dilemma of "fair compensation": a comparison with oocytes donation (OD)

Egg donation is strictly regulated where practiced in EU countries, must be non-commercial, and is a main reason for CBRC within Europe (Shenfield et al., 2010). Here also, issues and concerns of commercialization and exploitation of women are often raised, similarly to the case of surrogacy. In the EU, gametes must be donated, not paid by definition, as indeed both terms are actually contradictory (Shenfield and Steele, 1995), but compensation is not totally forbidden in several countries. The dilemma resides in the definition of a "fair" or "proportionate" compensation. In a recent study, we analyzed the motivations and characteristics of egg donors in 11 EU countries (Pennings et al., 2014). Five categories of motives were retained with the following results: pure altruism, 48%; mixed altruism plus financial benefit, 38%; 11% of women declared they donated for "pure(ly) financial benefit"; while a few declared their motivation was altruism plus own treatment, or "pure own treatment". The latter relates to the case of "egg sharing", where women agree to give some of their oocytes to another in need when they themselves go through IVF. In the private sector, this "egg sharing" often means a financial benefit by a cost reduction for the woman going through IVF if she donates some of her oocytes to another woman in need, and this is allowed in Europe – in Poland and the UK. The study showed that financial compensation helps to persuade some women to donate, and motivation to donate was further influenced by age (the older, the more altruistic), education (the higher educated, the more altruistic), and finally the amount of compensation (the lower, the more altruistic). Importantly, all monies were corrected by a Purchasing Power Parity analysis, in order to compare the economic benefit of the compensation in the 11 countries sampled through a common criterion.

It is known that the intended parent(s)' payment for commercial surrogacy with its contractual basis in the USA, or lower resource countries like India or Thailand, varies a lot, although there is little comparative data on sums changing hands, bar some press articles. By contrast, there is strict regulation in Greece and the UK, but those countries still face the difficulty of defining what is proportionate and fair compensation, in order not to entice and possibly coerce poorer women to take a risk on behalf of the intended parents. It would be very interesting to gather similar financial data for prospective surrogates, in order to further assess claims that surrogacy is "totally unethical" as an automatic abuse of women's dignity, either per se or by "buying/renting their womb". Such research would serve two purposes: first, finding out how many women define themselves in different countries according to the three categories from the European egg donors study (altruism, mixed altruism plus financial benefit, or pure financial benefit); and second, to agree on evidence-based policy, both nationally and internationally, according to what is best in order to support the autonomous choice of women undertaking surrogacy.

Whether the law offers sufficient ethical protection to surrogates may be further discussed by using the UK example.

Can legislation be a barrier to exploitation? The UK example

The Surrogacy Arrangement Act was passed by the UK Parliament in 1985,[2] making advertising, brokering, and profit-making by third parties a criminal offence. Since 1990, couples have been eligible for a parental order (PO) if married, domiciled in the UK, and at least one of them is a genetic parent; if the child's home is with the commissioning parents, the request is made within six months of the child's birth, valid consent was established, and only "reasonable expenses" – one of the very vexed questions – have been paid. From 2008, Part 3 of the HFE Act amends the Surrogacy Arrangements Act 1985 and makes new provisions, enabling "civil partners" to apply, as can unmarried opposite-sex couples or same-sex couples not in a civil partnership. The other provisions relating to PO remain the same as the existing provisions of the 1990 Act. Furthermore, the 2010 Regulations make clear that the "welfare of the child" would be a paramount consideration in any court decision.

It has been difficult to obtain accurate data from the last 30 years in which surrogacy has been legal in the UK, especially concerning the amount of surrogates' compensation. But a study of the number of PO issued by the UK courts has made very interesting reading (Crawshaw, Blyth, and van den Akker, 2012). In that study, a sharp increase in PO was noted from 2008 onwards: before 2008 they numbered 40–50 a year, but 73 PO were recorded in both 2008 and 2009; 75 in 2010; and 133 in 2011. Furthermore, the study highlights initial discrepancies between the figures supplied by the UK surrogacy agencies and the number of court orders issued until 2007, with a change to a very good match after 2007. In the years 2010–2012, the number of PO issued from surrogacy performed abroad were respectively 20 from India, 16 from the USA, and four from the Ukraine, out of a total of 190.

While the law has allowed many couples to go through satisfactory arrangements at home in the UK, some still go abroad, where the process of finding a surrogate may take less time, and where "brokers" rather than non-profit agencies may facilitate the process. This represents a small proportion of intended parents from the figures mentioned above, so surrogacy CBRC is not a common event. Nevertheless, this has led to complications when the commissioning parents return to the UK with a child, and to disproportionate political and sociological attention focusing on the immigration of the child thus conceived. Indeed, after noting some of the difficulties of British parents returning to the UK with a child conceived abroad, the British Home Office UK Border Agency issued guidance on "Inter-country surrogacy and the Immigration Rules" in 2009. This guidance explains that "with regards to visa applications, the United Kingdom recognizes surrogacy in India so long as it meets the conditions set out by the UK Human Fertilisation and Embryology Act 2008" and highlights not only the necessity "for a child to be treated in law as the child of a couple [it is necessary] to be genetically related to at least one of the commissioning couple", but also stresses the ethical concern that "no money other than reasonably incurred expenses has been paid in respect of the surrogacy arrangement". The term "reasonably" refers again to the constant dilemma of the proportionality of compensation or payment to surrogates, especially from low-income countries, and is left to the appreciation of the courts.

In general, the Border Agency also advises that the intended parents should try to obtain accurate information about their own national situation before embarking on the process, and that known legal problems or possible conflicts with the law in the home country should be explained to the patients. Indeed, there are now legal firms specializing in specific legal advice on surrogacy, international or otherwise in the UK.

It also appears that there may be fewer conflicts when parents return to a country where surrogacy is legal rather than where it is illegal (Brunet et al., 2013), as discussed below.

Some legal problems when intended parents return to their country

We illustrate here some of the legal dilemmas encountered by European "intended parents" who have obtained surrogacy abroad. The first two involve same-sex parents: a Spanish male married couple, and one from Belgium. The Spanish couple had twins born by egg donation and surrogacy in California in 2006, and a pre-birth judgment issued by a local court, but their consulate refused to issue visas to return to Spain. This conundrum was eventually resolved in 2011, after the Spanish Ministry of Justice weighed the interests of the children versus the interests of the Spanish government, which prohibits surrogacy. At the time, the Spanish ministry stressed the need to obtain a judgment in the host country court for the legal validity of the birth certificate, and to check that the contract for surrogacy was entered into "without fraud, overreaching or exploitation of the surrogate mother". With regards to the Belgian same-sex couple, they also had twins through a Californian surrogate: the Belgium High Court would only allow one (genetic) father on their birth certificate, rather than two as in the USA, and asked the non-biological father to adopt the children.

As surrogacy is forbidden in France, some French couples commission a surrogate in Belgium, who will then deliver "under X" in France, while the intended father can "recognize" the child before delivery. In such cases, Belgian clinicians report few problems when caring for patients from other countries, although some practices were modified, such as asking for advance payment, providing all appointments in one day, or providing interpreters (Brunet et al., 2013). Other French couples commission surrogacy in the USA, and an especially lengthy case is that of the Mennesson family, with their twins conceived by surrogacy in California in 2000.[3] The parents went through years of legal battle in order to obtain French citizenship for their children, which culminated on April 6, 2011, when France's highest court – the Court of Cassation – refused this, with the possible ensuing obstacles to school registration, healthcare access, and inheritance. Finally, in 2014, the twins' parents' status and nationality was resolved in the European Court of Human Rights (ECt HR). The Court stated that "totally prohibiting the establishment of a relationship between a father and his biological children born following surrogacy arrangements abroad was in breach of the (Human Rights) Convention" and that there was no violation of Article 8 (right to respect for private and family life) of the European Convention on Human Rights concerning the applicants' right in respect of their family life; but there was a violation of Article 8 concerning the children's right in respect of their private life. Thus the ECt HR ordered France to recognize and provide French citizenship to children born to surrogate mothers abroad, even though surrogacy is illegal in France. The decision was widely celebrated as a recognition of the "best interests of the child" standard, and a sign of progress in France for such children left in legal limbos, although one commentator worried that this might yet further entrench national positions not to accept surrogacy on their territory (Bala, 2014).

Conclusion

The legal puzzle of CBRC with third parties may be solved nationally or internationally, such as in Europe with the above French example. Advice may be available in the commissioning parents' country, such as that provided by the UK Border Agency.

Furthermore, the Indian legislation which is to be presented to Parliament in the near future (ART (Regulation) Bill, 2015) provides new specific conditions for surrogacy in India, which should help to clarify the path of commissioning parents. They will need to appoint a local guardian if not resident in the country and arrange appropriate insurance for the surrogate, who must be aged between 21 and 35.

Nevertheless, recourse to the law can be a lengthy process after the facts, thus taking a long time to alleviate the respective families' anxieties. Gathering facts and furthering research allows transparency, an ethical duty to patients, and society at large. One suggestion is gathering more data on the motivations of surrogates internationally in order to have more transparency and evidence on which to establish ethical non-commercial systems which will not fall prey to the criticism tainting the whole field of "gestating for another", as the French call surrogacy. Thus, the plans of the Hague Conference on private international law, which produced a "Study of legal parentage and the issues arising from international surrogacy arrangements" in April 2014, and stated the desirability of further work, are welcome. The document highlights the (legal) "paradox" where "the internal laws of many states concerning the establishment and contestation of legal parentage have been very influenced by social, scientific and demographic changes", and the modern medical technologies, such as surrogacy, which challenge genetic "certainty" and allow parental "intention" to be distinct entities, whether by gamete donation or surrogacy.

While there is a corpus of evidence on gamete donation, there is a need for more evidence and data concerning the frequency and conditions of surrogacy, especially in low resource countries, the amount of compensation, and other transactions, both for the surrogates and intermediaries when they exist. From acceptance of the technique to emotive press titles, the main questions remain the informed nature of the surrogates' consent, the possible commercialization of their body, and the nature and extent of their compensation. Can a fair and ethical non-commercial system exist while waiting for uterus transplants to become routine, which may take many years (Brännström et al., 2015)? Can the offspring's legal status, parentage, and nationality ensure that the "welfare of the (future) child", or best interests of the born child, are maximized, and at what (ethical) costs? Where do we turn when recommendations and guidelines to promote professional responsibility and respect for women's autonomy are seriously challenged, especially through economic pressure (Shetty, 2012)? Failing effective action by medical professional associations and/or licensing authorities, only the law, with its symbolic and coercive strong arm, may then, we hope, provide the solution. Whilst Thailand has recently reacted to scandal surrounding surrogacy by a ban of the technique (Sharp, 2014), it is encouraging that India's legislators are following this arduous path in the case of surrogacy, but it remains to be seen when the ART Bill will become law, and what means of implementation will be enacted.

When intended parents plan to go abroad, they often have recourse to internet sites for information (Shenfield et al., 2010). With this knowledge, ESHRE's guide to good clinical practice in CBRC was actually linked, when published, to many sites, including the UK National Patients Association, several European statutory authorities, and several national fertility societies, as well as the websites of the Canadian and Australian statutory authorities (Shenfield, 2012). In the UK, some legal firms have specialized in advising intended parents going abroad for surrogacy, and this should be commended. However, it is more difficult for European citizens residing in countries where the technique is banned to find a path where ethics and law are balanced when going abroad. Whether this may be a reason for such countries to accept surrogacy remains to be seen.

Notes

1 HFE Act, 2008. Available from: http://www.legislation.gov.uk/ukpga/2008/22/contents
2 Surrogacy Arrangement Act, 1985. Available from: http://www.legislation.gov.uk/ukpga/1985/49/contents
3 *Mennesson vs France* and *Labassee vs France*. Available from: http://www.hudoc.echr.coe.int/webservices/content/pdf/003-4804617-5854908

References

ART (Regulation) Draft Bill (Sept. 30, 2015), Available from: www.nic.in.

Bala N (2014), The hidden costs of the ECt HR Surrogacy Decision, *Yale Journal of International Law on line*, vol 40, pp.10–19.

Brännström M, Johannesson L, Bokström H, Kvarnström N, Mölne J, Dahm-Kähler P, Enskog A, Milenkovic M, Ekberg J, Diaz-Garcia C, Gäbel M, Hanafy A, Hagberg H, Olausson M, and Nilsson L (2015), Live Birth after uterine transplant, *The Lancet*, 385:607–16.

Brunet L, Carruthers J, Davaki K, King D, Marzo C, and Mcclandless J (2013), A comparative study on the Regime of Surrogacy in EU Member States, Directorate General for Internal Policies, Policies Department C: Citizens' Rights and Constitutional Affairs, Legal and Parliamentary Affairs, European Parliament, Brussels.

Crawshaw M, Blyth E, and van den Akker O (2012), The changing profile of surrogacy in the UK – Implications for national and international policy and practice. *Journal of Social Welfare and Family Law*, 34(3):267–277.

Commission of the European Communities (2008), Proposal for a Directive of the European Parliament and of the Council on the application of patients' rights in cross-border healthcare, Presented by the European Commission on 2 July 2008, Copyright: European Communities, 2008; Directorate-General for Health and Consumers, European Commission – B-1049, Brussels.

Commission of the European Communities (2006), 2006/86/EC of 24 October 2006 implementing Directive 2004/23/EC of the European Parliament and of the Council as regards traceability requirements, notification of serious adverse reactions and events and certain technical requirements for the coding, processing, preservation, storage and distribution of human tissues and cells.

Dickens B (1997), Interfaces of assisted reproduction ethics and law, in *Ethical Dilemmas in Assisted Reproduction*, F Shenfield and C Sureau (eds), New York and London: Parthenon.

FIGO Committee for the Ethical Aspects of Human Reproduction and Women's Health (2008), Surrogacy, *International Journal of Gynaecology & Obstetrics*, 102(3):312–313.

Pennings G, de Wert G, Shenfield F, Cohen J, Tarlatzis B, and Devroey P, on behalf of ESHRE Task Force on Ethics and Law 15 (2008): Cross-border reproductive care. *Human Reproduction*, 23(10):2,182–2,184.

Pennings G., J. de Mouzon, F. Shenfield, A.P. Ferraretti, T. Mardesic, A. Ruiz, and V. Goossens (2014). Socio-demographic and fertility-related characteristics and motivations of oocyte donors in eleven European countries, *Human Reproduction*, 29(5): 1076–1089.

Sharp J (2014), Thai parliament votes to outlaw commercial surrogacy. Bionews, December 2014. Available from: http://www.bionews.org.uk/page_473990.asp

Shenfield F and Steele SJ (1995), A gift is a gift is a gift, or why gametes donors should not be paid. *Human Reproduction*, (10):253–254.

Shenfield F, Pennings G, Cohen J, Devroey P, de Wert G, and Tarlatzis B, on behalf of ESHRE Task Force on Ethics and Law (2005): Surrogacy, *Human Reproduction*, 20(10):2,705–2,707.

Shenfield F, de Mouzon J, Pennings G, Ferraretti AP, Andersen AN, de Wert G, and Goossens V (2010). Cross-Border Reproductive Care in Six European Countries. *Human Reproduction*, 25(6):1,361– 1,368.

Shenfield F (2012), Implementing a cross border reproductive care (CBRC) good practice guide: Perspectives from the ESHRE Cross Border Reproductive Care Taskforce, *Reproductive biomedicine online*, 23:665–676.

Shetty P (2012), India's unregulated surrogacy industry, *The Lancet*, 380:1,633–1,634.

11 'All one needs is a credit card'

Transnational surrogacy in India on weblogs and in documentaries

Karen Hvidtfeldt

Lila, the 'million rupee baby', was born in 2009 at the Akanksha Infertility Clinic in the small town of Anand in the Indian state Gujerat. This clinic became known worldwide after Dr. Nayana Patel appeared in the *Oprah Winfrey Show* episode 'Wombs for Rent' in 2007, where she branded surrogacy as 'India's gift to the world'. On her weblog (millionrupeebaby.blogspot.com), Lila's mum shares the pain of being infertile, the many considerations before the difficult decision of choosing an Indian surrogacy clinic, the worries during the long-distance pregnancy, and later the joy of parenthood (Figure 11.1).

No exact measurements exist regarding the extent of surrogacy in India. Sociologist Amrita Pande documented that more than 100 surrogate babies were born at the Armaan clinic[1] in 2013. Since its opening in 2004, surrogates at this clinic have given birth to more than 600 babies; the children have been passed on to couples residing in more than 29 foreign countries (Pande, 2014: 19). The Mumbai-based fertility bank, Surrogacy India, claims that more than 295 surrogate babies have been born since it opened in 2007. Of those cases, 90% involved international clients and 40% were same-sex couples (Bhalla & Thapliyal, 2013). In 2014, *The Indian Express* estimated the current number of surrogacy cases in

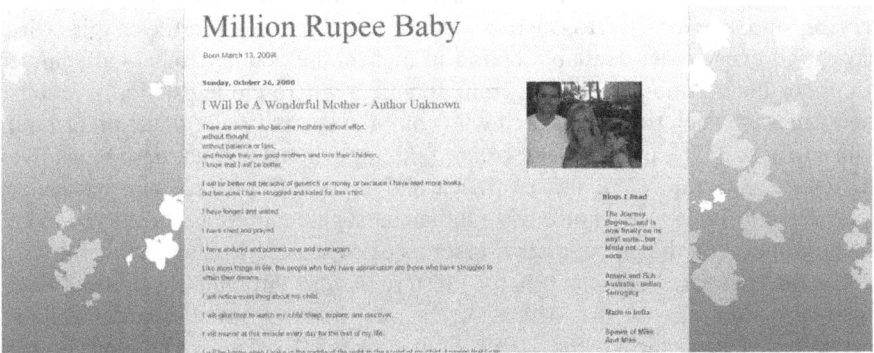

Figure 11.1 The weblog Million Rupee Baby shares the challenges and concerns of a couple going through transnational surrogacy

Source: http://millionrupeebaby.blogspot.dk/2008/10/i-will-be-wonderful-mother-author.html

India to be between 400 and 500, with about 30% involving international patients (Ghosh, 2014). Estimates of the number of Indian fertility clinics vary from 350 to over 3,000; a UN-backed study in July 2012 valued the surrogacy business at more than $400 million a year (Hochschild, 2009; Bhalla & Thapliyal, 2013).

Indian fertility clinics offer treatments and surrogacy services to both Indian and Western customers at prices that are very competitive to a Western market. This marketplace, where bodies and body parts are being priced and exchanged, has drawn attention from social science researchers and led to important ethnographic and sociological analyses. In this chapter, I offer analytical perspectives on narratives and discourses published in publicly available weblogs (blogs) that are held by Western parents and intended parents of Indian surrogate children, as well as documentaries on the subject that are produced by Western filmmakers. As a cultural studies scholar, I examine the media texts from a cultural studies perspective as social and cultural practices. Thus, I identify metaphors and study the arguments constructed by bloggers in order to make sense of the situation and legitimize the use of an Indian surrogate. I examine how the surrogates are presented and constructed, both from the point of view of the bloggers and as subjects in the documentaries, and argue that surrogacy overall is framed as a 'do-it-your-self project' within a neoliberal framework of understanding (Hvidtfeldt, 2015a, 2015b; Kroløkke & Pant, 2012; Rose, 2005, 2007; Vora, 2009). However, my aim is also to point out that the blogs and documentaries offer nuanced insights into the understandings and motivations of involved parties. Fixed identities are resisted and changing understandings of kinship and relatedness develop in the narratives while surrogacy is considered, negotiated, and acted out by the individual surrogates, the intended and commissioning parents, the fertility clinics, and the intermediaries.[2]

Surrogacy on weblogs

Publicly available on the Internet, there are numerous blogs on the subject of surrogacy in India (Figures 11.1–3).[3] The blog authors are Western parents or intended parents carrying out transnational fertility treatments involving the services of one or more surrogate mothers in India. Some are infertile couples who have tried every other available option in their home country; others are single people or male same-sex couples from countries where the legislation prohibits their access to such treatments, and who combine sperm or egg donation or both with surrogacy. The intended and commissioning parents behind these blogs live in Europe, Australia, or North America and often do not have any particular connection to India. The choice of an Indian surrogate mother is considered to be the best option on the global market in terms of cost, expertise, and availability.[4]

The Internet plays a crucial role for Western parents throughout a transnational surrogacy process, as the extensive use of Internet-based communication technology reduces the adverse effects of geographical distance. The blogs reveal that intended parents from the West seek out clinics on the Internet, eventually following the Indian surrogate's pregnancy check-ups on Skype and regularly communicating with the doctors and surrogates through digital media. Blogs have

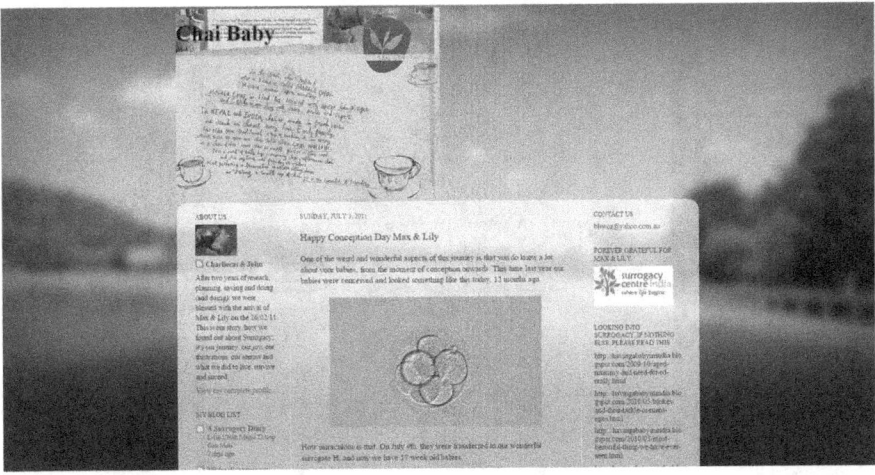

Figure 11.2a The weblog Chai Baby celebrates the conception day of twins carried by a surrogate in India

Source: http://havingababyinindia.blogspot.dk/2011/07/happy-conception-day-max-lily.html

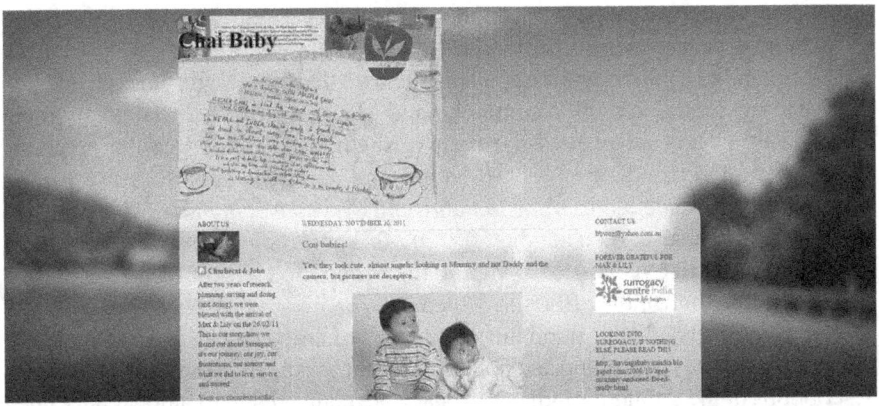

Figure 11.2b Chai Baby follows the children's development and also shares knowledge on Indian culture, e.g. the traditions of Masala Chai

Source: http://havingababyinindia.blogspot.dk/2011/11/con-babies.html

been a decisive factor in the professionalization of the intended parents, who share information and experiences worldwide within seconds. The bloggers often express a feeling of solidarity towards each other and an obligation to disseminate relevant factual information about the clinics, their procedures, and how to deal with Indian and domestic authorities. Opinions among the intended and commissioning parents are also exchanged and negotiated on the Internet. Desire, joy, and despair are circulated between people (who in many cases never meet in

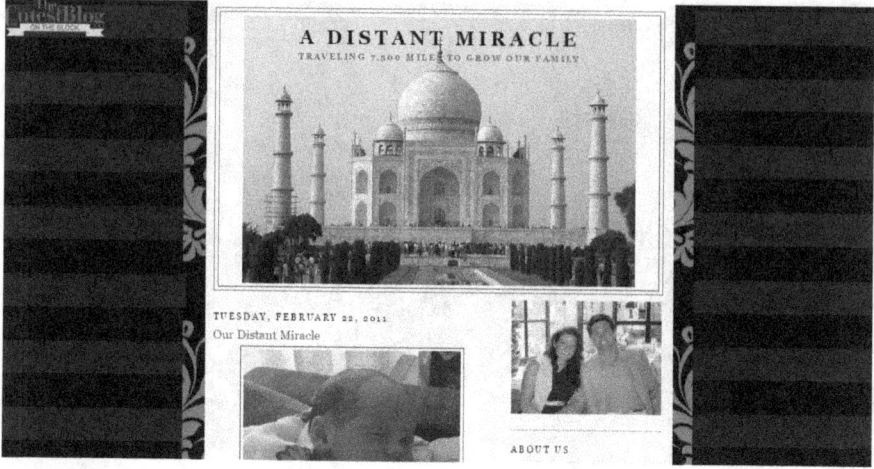

Figure 11.3 On the blog A DISTANT MIRACLE the Taj Mahal at the same time represents India and symbolizes the enormous importance of becoming parents

Source: http://adistantmiracle.blogspot.dk/2011/02/our-distant-miracle.html

person) in order to make transnational surrogacy seem like a natural and respectable practice within an environment of global possibilities.

The intended parents narrate a pregnancy that they are not physically experiencing in the virtual community and share a visual chronicle of their journey: ultrasound pictures of the fetus' growth, 'belly shots' of the pregnant surrogate, and portraits of new-born babies and children. The blogs use names such as *Million Rupee Baby, Made in India*, and *Procreated in India*, with strategic cover images such as Indian handicraft (*Taj Ma Baby*), colorful sarees (*Christmas Eve Boys*) or tourist venues to downplay the economic element of the surrogacy process and dramatize the efforts involved.

Intended parents often position the surrogate mothers as unreal, supernatural, and magical, sometimes describing and portraying them as 'angels'. These narratives and descriptions of the setting for Indian surrogacy are compared to traditional fairy tales where the hero meets a number of complications before succeeding and living happily ever after, and borrow from magical realism, in that bloggers often characterize their journey as an adventure in a distant and foreign land. Humor, irony, and a variety of metaphoric frames are used to express the intense emotions that follow the process, at the same time supporting the reconstruction of a neoliberal logic.

Online parenthood: globalization and neoliberalism

Anthropologist Emily Martin studies how common understandings of women's bodies and reproductive systems are shaped by the language and metaphors used to describe them (Martin, 2001). In blogs about surrogate motherhood, the neoliberal frame of mind is highlighted as the surrogate's ability and right to dispose of her own body, including her right to make money on surrogate motherhood as a service. The commissioning parents, however, downplay the money they pay, instead highlighting the mental effort that parenthood has 'cost' them. The blogs document these struggles and legitimize the children's creation stories.

Surrogacy bloggers often define themselves and each other as particularly dedicated parents by virtue of what they have endured. In their blogs, the journey metaphor is used to dramatize the emotional investment over the financial investment made by intended parents, and the physical pain of labor is used as a metaphor for the challenges that prospective parents of surrogate children face. Common metaphors include references to not only their 'journey' but also to the surrogacy process as a 'marathon', which signals both the length of the process and the emotional strength required for transnational surrogacy.[5] Surrogacy bloggers argue that parents who experience infertility have invested more than those who become pregnant without problems. Even though parents of surrogate children have not experienced the physical pregnancy, they have felt and lived through pain comparable with an actual birth. By accepting this argument, they become legitimate parents, despite not having gone through pregnancy and in many cases lacking genetic relation to the child.

The bloggers stress both their own and the surrogate mother's active efforts as significant, and argue that their own intentionality is crucial in establishing kinship with the child. Martin argues that metaphors used to describe the female body and reproduction during the twentieth century were influenced by the industrial society (e.g. efficiency, regularity), and that they have since moved into what she describes as a theoretical framework of chaos, where the unpredictable and flexible count as ideals (Martin, 2001). Similarly, the bloggers have developed metaphors that reflect late-modern ideals in the era of globalization. For example, Megan celebrated the global community and welcomed the transnational opportunities made available through web communications:

> So, here we have an egg donor from South Africa, a surrogate in India and a couple in Australia making a family. Wow. It is such an honour to be the instigator of this process and make friends with people from across the world, who only have our best interests at heart.[6]

Tracy compared her experience of the Indian surrogacy process with a sports team, also using late-modern business management rhetoric in which coaching, project management, and team building are key words:

> Anyone pursuing surrogacy should know that it is the ultimate team effort.
> - M is the captain – the glue (literally) that holds us all together
> - I am the quarterback – in charge of distributing the ball (or eggs, if you will)
> - B is on special teams – usually on the sidelines, but an indispensable part of the team
> - Dr. Patel is the coach – writing the play book and leading us all to victory
>
> We have learned to trust in and have created a lifelong bond with our new teammates. Although we all have different tasks we all share the same goal.[7]

Megan chose to present her 'team' as solely driven by altruistic motives, while Tracy highlighted the more emotional aspects of the partnership. In her quote, the surrogate mother (M) stars as 'captain', and the doctors become 'coaches', while the recipient couple takes on more peripheral positions.

Thus, globalization is both the basis for the Internet-based community of bloggers and a theme in the construction of virtual motherhood. The bloggers at the same time identify and distance the act of transnational surrogacy from a commercial transaction of buying or hiring a womb by virtue of these metaphors of global connection. The relationship with the Indian surrogates is narrated as a late-modern global teamwork where all stakeholders are granted agency and respectability. Both the childless Westerners and the poor citizens in India are transformed into active entrepreneurs and presented as rational subjects who deliberately make their own choices using neoliberal logic. While the commissioning parents place emphasis on the opportunity to become parents, the surrogate mothers prioritize economic mobility (Krøløkke & Pant, 2012). Surrogacy is described as an emotional investment for the intended parents; the journey metaphor (and the fairy-tale resemblance) is used to underline the intensity of the process.

The blogs and the digital technology compensate for the lack of embodiment and proximity, as well as the feeling of isolation and loneliness often experienced by commissioning parents who are expecting children through surrogacy. They blur the line between being pregnant and not pregnant in the flow of reproductive fluids, body parts, intentions, and desires, and the social and genetic relationships are also blurred. In several cases, bloggers refer to each other as 'blog family' and express the feeling of being more closely connected to peers in the blog world than they are to their biological families (DasGupta and Dasgupta, 2010, 2011).

Documentaries: *Google Baby* and *Made in India*

The documentaries *Google Baby* (Frank, 2009)[8] and *Made in India* (Haimowitz & Sinha, 2010)[9] circulate online and are often referenced in surrogacy blogs. Like the blogs, these documentaries place transnational reproduction treatments in a neoliberal frame of understanding, and they rewrite and legitimize the stories as recognizable liberation projects. In *Made in India*, the surrogate mother frees Lisa from her infertile body; in *Google Baby*, Doron and other gay men gain access to parenthood though surrogacy, while the grandmother achieves a prominent position as care provider. The gay, childless man and the heterosexual, childless woman are presented as legitimate consumers in a transnational reproductive economy. Not only the infertile Westerners, but also the egg donor and the Indian surrogate are understood as entrepreneurs, consciously acting in a free market. Egg donation and surrogacy also make it possible for the US egg donor, Kat, and Indian surrogate mothers to take positions as modern subjects and consumers.

In *Google Baby*, the neoliberal framework is initially linked with the sexual liberation of Western women in the 1960s, when the contraceptive pill:

turned sex into an act independent of the risk of pregnancy. Today, technology has turned 'making a baby' into an act independent of sex. And globalization is making it affordable. All one needs is a credit card.

In this quote, the pill and sexual liberation are presented as equal with ART and further associated with global consumer culture. *Google Baby* furthermore highlights that it is favorable that surrogate motherhood does not require special skills or 'particular training'. This is also evident in other scenes in *Google Baby*, such as when Doron normalizes the outsourcing of pregnancies to India as part of a general trend that also takes place among the big IT companies: 'I have a high tech background and outsourcing to India is very trendy right now' (Frank, 2009).

In line with the neoliberal philosophy, the main characters in these two films achieve citizenship through parenthood and consumption. In *Made in India*, we see Lisa busy arranging her 'baby shower' and how she stages herself as mother-to-be through the exchange of gifts and consumption. This also applies to Doron, a gay man who achieves parenthood through surrogacy and reinstalls what the American theorist Lisa Duggan refers to as heteronormative structures (Duggan, 2003).

In *Google Baby*, the main character, Doron, personifies and embodies globalization, mobility, and agency, as he travels around the world on airplane, by car, and in a rickshaw. He lives in an openly homosexual relationship and occupies a familiar position as he and his partner become parents through ART and transnational surrogacy. However, quite traditionally, it is his mother who stays home with the baby while he works, and they keep in touch on their mobile phones. He meets with his daughter's egg donor on Skype, allowing the donor to be part of her life to some extent, and he shows his clients how they can meet and choose egg donors online on a clinic's website.

Made in India and *Google Baby* show how infertile individuals make choices to optimize their possibility of having children. The surrogates in *Google Baby* are mainly presented as passive and uninformed, as they patiently await the progress of pregnancy and the decisions made for them by other stakeholders in the clinic. However, the egg donor, Kat, decides on her own to repeatedly sell her eggs, and in *Made in India*, Aasia is positioned as a modern woman, who makes up her own mind to be a surrogate, even without the consent of her husband. At first she laughed with disbelief at the possibility of becoming pregnant 'without having a relationship', but once she understood the basic principle of ART, she signed the agreements without her husband's consent. Once he realized that she was pregnant, it was too late to undo the act. Aasia said that she was 'a little scared' when she learned of the twin pregnancy, but was helped by her faith. She was told that the children would be going abroad, but she does not seem particularly concerned about the surrogate children. Her main concern is her earnings and what she can do for the children that she has at home. Aasia avoids being seen as an exploited victim. She gains respect by acting as an entrepreneur and highlights that she is a surrogate for the sake of her own children.

For Lisa and Aasia in *Made in India* and for Diksha in *Google Baby*, the identity of motherhood is considered a dominant and respectable position. The emotions connected to motherhood – love, desire, and hope – are used to naturalize and legitimize their choices and actions. *Made in India* shows how the paradoxical relationship between the feeling of agency or no agency, choice and no choice are negotiated: in Lisa's understanding of her own situation, she has an absence of choice; this is her last and only option to have a child, and she:

> just can't imagine being without kids. I've wanted to be a mother since I was about 25 years of age, and here I am turning 40 … I am heartfelt. I am determined. This is my dream. This is what I need to be whole.

Like Lisa, Aasia uses motherhood as an argument. Rather than framing her activity as a surrogate in the neoliberal terms of selling or renting out her womb, she states that her concern is first and foremost as a mother: 'Everything I do, I do for the children, for their happiness' – here referring to her children at home.

Meanwhile, being an infertile woman is an important part of Lisa's identity, as described in the previously mentioned blogs. Lisa's painful injections are put on display, as are the many stressful situations she goes through at home and in India. In comparison, remarkably few of the surrogate mother Aasia's treatments are shown. She seems calm compared to Lisa, who (in her own words) is 'kind of freaking out'. Lisa views herself as a diagnosed patient, but she and Brian also identify themselves as 'fighters'. They feel forced into a 'reproductive exile' of sorts, because of the high costs of fertility treatments in the US: 'In the US, if you're struggling to have a child, you have to be a lawyer or a doctor to afford this. It's not fair.' The position of economic marginality is highlighted as a defense against less respectable positions, as Lisa and Brian are seen negotiating at the clinic in the same way as at the local Indian marketplace. They are also shown walking around town as tourists, expressing their intentions of maybe also going to see the Taj Mahal. At home, they are directly confronted as villains, as they take part in a talk show on NBC and afterwards defend themselves against hate talk on the Internet.

Discussion and conclusions

The blogs show how the Western intended and commissioning parents of surrogate children legitimize an entrepreneurial way of thinking and acting. They construct narratives that downplay the unpleasant fact of the very unequal levels of privilege within transnational surrogacy, and the Indian surrogate is granted respectability on the intended parent's conditions. Surrogates are presented as respectable angel-like mother figures in a fairy-tale narrative, or as stakeholders in a professional business relationship. Affect and humor are used as rhetorical strategies to legitimize surrogacy as an acceptable way of creating kinship within the neoliberal frame of thought.

In their article 'Motherhood Jeopardized', Sayantani DasGupta and Shamita Das Dasgupta critique the altruistic rhetoric in popular media and in the international marketing materials used by Indian fertility clinics, arguing that the surrogate is often positioned as being led by altruistic motives. They stress that not only is economic exploitation at stake, but the 'very rhetoric of global gestational surrogacy in India reflects a sort of cultural and physically invasive colonialization' (DasGupta and Dasgupta, 2010: 139). According to DasGupta and Dasgupta, this forms the basis for the 'othering' of the gestational mothers, who are 'not just made different from the women who hire them, but from the fetuses they carry as well' (DasGupta and Dasgupta, 2010: 142), with reference to the publishing of belly shots and ultrasound images. My readings of the blogs and documentaries support these arguments.

However, I also wish to resist 'depictions of women who become surrogates as powerless victims in need of aid' as stressed by Daisy Deomampo, who 'contend[s] that reliance on the image of the oppressed surrogate neglects the local voices and perspectives long sought by ethnographers and feminists' (Deomampo, 2013). In the blogs and documentaries, individuals frame their understanding of surrogacy within a neoliberal setting, wherein each person is in charge of his or her own life and body and able to take responsibility for getting the most out of available opportunities (Rose, 2005). Thus, it is – within a neoliberal discourse – the choice of the egg donor if she wants to 'deal' with her eggs; the surrogate mother can also make her own choices, and correspondingly it is the choice of the childless whether they will accept their condition or do what is necessary to change the situation.

The blogs and documentaries furthermore underline that Indian surrogates and Western prospective parents operate on very unequal terms. While the economically privileged intended parents travel across continents several times during the process, the Indian surrogates typically do not leave their local environment, do not speak English, and do not have Internet access. Like access to ART, agency on the Internet is unevenly distributed; there is a clear hierarchy and direction of power in the global movements. Indian surrogate mothers do not have the same opportunities to influence their situation as the Western intended parents, for whom writing blogs and viewing films are just two of many ways in which to develop and exchange views.

The narratives also reveal that all parties involved in the process add to new and changing understandings of what kinship and relatedness means in a globalized society. The narratives found on the blogs and in the documentaries voice the concrete challenges of individual agents of transnational surrogacy and offer insights to the ambivalent and diverse understandings of kinship and relatedness that have followed the globalization of medical and technological reproduction. In the documentaries, not only the commissioning parents, but also several surrogates emphasize that genetic kinship is essential compared to gestational or social connections. In *Made in India*, the 'natural' bonds between parents and their 'own' children are promoted in various ways, and Lisa points at the genetic connection as being exclusive: 'These are my genetic children. I should not have to go through this' (Haimowitz & Sinha, 2010). Yet, critical perspectives are also established. The documentary presents clear oppositions between the very large Americans (double XL) and the thin Indians (often seen begging in the streets). Thus, visual and verbal arguments are blended as are the questions of privilege and kinship, as the film questions whether the rights that Lisa and Brian claim over the children are actually based upon genetic connections or rather on the economic superiority made manifest through their large bodies. Surrogates, parents, and donors transform emotions (pain, love) into relatedness and highlight understandings of kinship based on mixtures of genetic and social relations – virtual contact on the blogs and physical contact in the clinics. The documentaries' critical views of the commissioning parents' motives are based on Doron's clients' assumed lack of emotional engagement.

As the title of *Google Baby* suggests, the child becomes a commodity comparable to other goods that are often purchased on the Internet. Technology has freed reproduction from sex, globalization has made surrogacy economically feasible, and the credit card makes it easy. However, the film itself and the analysis of surrogacy blogs have shown that transnational surrogacy holds challenges that do take more than a credit card to solve. The Internet has opened a global market of ART and surrogacy and given Western intended parents the possibility to communicate their experiences. Neoliberal structures obviously include the human body and the process of reproduction. National legislation no longer restricts transnational interactions in this area and transnational negotiations and cooperation are highly relevant and needed.

Notes

1 Fictitious name.
2 My work is a part of a research project founded by the Danish research council from 2010–2014: '(Trans)Formations of Kinship: Travelling in Search of Relatedness' (KinTra), a group of researchers working on different areas of fertility treatments, fertility travel, transnational adoption, and transformations of family and kinship. The project questions how ART interacts with understandings of kinship, including the importance of new media and social networking sites, which not only speed up communication between different stakeholders but also create new ways to express and negotiate relatedness. Parts of this paper are also published in 'A Baby "Made in India"': Weblogs on Motherhood, Consumerism and Privilege in Transnational Surrogacy'. In J. L. Bordo, A. T. Demo, and C. Kroløkke (eds), *The Motherhood Business: Consumption, Communication, Privilege.* Tuscaloosa: University of Alabama Press (2015); in 'Documentaries on transnational surrogacy in India: Questions of privilege, respectability and kinship'. In *Critical Kinship*, C. Kroløkke, L. Myong, S. W. Adrian and Tine Tjørnhøj-Thomsen (eds), Rowman and Littlefield International (2015), and in Scandinavian anthologies and scholarly journals.
3 I have followed about 20 weblogs since 2009, all dealing with the specific subject of surrogacy in India. Some of the weblogs are still active, but most are no longer updated, as the surrogacy process has ended.
4 In July 2013, the Indian government updated visa regulations and the process to obtain a specific surrogate visa now requires a valid (heterosexual) marriage certificate showing that parents have been married for at least two years and a formal letter from the home country stating that surrogacy is recognized and legal. This new regulation excludes all applicants from countries that do not officially recognize transnational surrogacy, the entire gay community, and singles coming from abroad. In response to these new restrictions in India, surrogacy destinations are opening in Mexico, Thailand, and Nepal, and thus the global market of surrogacy moves constantly. To maintain its competitive

edge in these emerging markets, the Indian government decided in 2014 to allow the import of frozen human embryos for artificial reproduction. This makes it more flexible and swift to bring in or ship human embryos that are prepared for implantation in the surrogate womb and might make the surrogacy experience in India more attractive for foreign couples.

5 Chai Baby, 'UPDATED: Blokes and Their Tackle or: Men's Egos Around Fertility Are as Fragile as Chooks Eggs with Calcium Deficiency', May 30, 2010. Available from: http://havingababyinindia.blogspot.com (accessed March 21, 2014).

6 Amani and Bob's Indian Surrogacy, 'Thunderbirds Are GO!,' September 28, 2008. Available from: http://amaniandbobsurrogacy.blogspot.com (accessed November 22, 2011).

7 Million Rupee Baby, 'Play Like a Champion Today', August 3, 2008. Available from: http://millionrupeebaby.blogspot.com (accessed November 22, 2011).

8 The documentary *Google Baby* follows Doron, a gay man from Israel, who is the father of a daughter born by a surrogate in the US. He wants to start a business servicing other gay couples who want to be parents, but are unable – or unwilling – to pay US prices for a surrogate mother. The narration follows him to the US, where he buys donor eggs and has them fertilized and sent to India, where surrogacy is more affordable. We meet Katherine, a 28-year-old American who has successfully donated eggs, and plans to donate again to help pay for the remodeling of her family's home. Doron travels to Anand in Gujarat, West India, where he seeks out the famous Dr. Nayana Patel (known from *Oprah Winfrey's* talk show) and enquires about the possibility of using Indian surrogates in her clinic.

9 *Made in India* tells the story of an American couple from San Antonio, Texas, Lisa and Brian Switzer, who sold their house to go to India for surrogacy services after seven years of infertility, stating that 'this is our one and final shot'. The medical tourism company, Planet Hospital, promised them an affordable solution in Mumbai, where the clinic Rutunda specializes in transnational surrogacy arrangements. The couple happily learns that 'their' surrogate is pregnant, and later, that she is expecting twins. They are, as Doron was, very engaged intended parents and follow every possible step of the surrogate's pregnancy process. The 27-year-old surrogate Aasia lives in a one-room house in a slum in Mumbai with her husband and their three children. Aasia was introduced to the fertility clinic by her sister-in-law, who follows her throughout the process. She is an unorthodox Muslim, and wears a burka mostly to hide her identity from the neighbors as she enters the fertility clinic to be implanted with Lisa and Brian's embryos.

References

Bhalla, N., Thapliyal, M. (2013). India Seeks to Regulate Its Booming 'Rent-A-Womb' Industry. Reuters, September 30, 2013. Available from: http://www.reuters.com/article/2013/09/30/us-india-surrogates-idUSBRE98T07F20130930 (accessed March 11, 2014).

DasGupta, S., Dasgupta, S. D. (2010). Motherhood jeopardized. In J. Maher and W. Chavkin (eds), *The Globalization of Motherhood: Deconstructions and reconstructions of biology and care*. New York: Routledge, pp. 131–153.

DasGupta, S., Dasgupta, S. D. (2011). Transnational Surrogacy, E-Motherhood, and Nation Building. In M. Moravec (ed.), *Motherhood Online*. Cambridge: Cambridge Scholars Publishing, pp. 283–311.

Deomampo, D. (2013). Transnational Surrogacy in India: Interrogating Power and Women's Agency. *Frontiers*, 34(3):167.

Duggan, L. (2003). *The twilight of equality? Neoliberalism, cultural politics, and the attack on democracy*. Boston: Beacon Press.

Frank, Z. B. (Writer). (2009). *Google Baby*. H. D. F. Brandcom Productions, Yes (Producer). Israel.

Ghosh, S. A. (2014). In Boost to Infertility Treatment, Government Allows Import of Frozen Embryos. *The Indian Express*, Available from: http://indianexpress.com/article/technology/science/in-boost-to-infertility-treatment-govt-allows-import-of-frozen-embryos/ (accessed 21 June, 2014).

Haimowitz, R., Sinha, V. (Writers). (2010). *Made in India*. C. A. E. Pictures & T. F. Fund (Producer). USA.

Hochschild, A. (2009). Childbirth at the Global Crossroads. *The American Prospect*, 20(8):25–28.

Hvidtfeldt, K. (2015a). A Baby 'Made in India': Motherhood, Consumerism, and Privilege in Transnational Surrogacy. In A. Demo, J. Borda and C. Kroløkke (eds), *The Motherhood Business: Consumption, Communication, and Privilege*. Tuscaloosa, AL: The University of Alabama Press.

Hvidtfeldt, K. (2015b). Documentaries on Transnational Surrogacy in India: Questions of Privilege, Respectability and Kinship. In C. Kroløkke, L. Myong, S. Adrian and T. Tjørnhøj-Thomsen (eds), *Critical Kinship*. London: Rowman & Littlefield International.

Kroløkke, C., Pant, S. (2012). 'I only need her uterus': Neo-liberal Discourses on Transnational Surrogacy. *NORA: Nordic Journal of Women's Studies*, 20(4):233.

Martin, E. (2001). *The woman in the body: a cultural analysis of reproduction* (Vol. Rev. ed.). Boston: Beacon Press.

Pande, A. (2014). *Wombs in labor: transnational commercial surrogacy in India*. New York: Columbia University Press.

Rose, N. (2005). *Powers of freedom: reframing political thought*. Cambridge: Cambridge University Press.

Rose, N. (2007). *The politics of life itself: biomedicine, power and subjectivity in the twenty-first century*. Princeton, NJ: Princeton University Press.

Vora, K. (2009). Indian transnational surrogacy and the commodification of vital energy. *Subjectivity*, 28(1):266–278.

Winfrey, O. (2007). Journey to Parenthood. Available from: http://www.oprah.com/world/Wombs-for-Rent (accessed December 2, 2011).

Weblogs

Amani and Bob's Indian Surrogacy. http://amaniandbobsurrogacy.blogspot.com (accessed November 22, 2011).

Chai Baby. http://havingababyinindia.blogspot.com (accessed March 21, 2014).

Christmas Eve Boys. http://christmaseveboys.blogspot.com/ (accessed November 21, 2011).

CocoaMasala. http://cocoamasala.blogspot.com/ (accessed November 21, 2013).

Million Rupee Baby. http://millionrupeebaby.blogspot.com (accessed March 17, 2014).

Procreated in India. http://procreatedinindia.blogspot.com (accessed March 17, 2014).

Taj Ma Baby. http://tajmababy.blogspot.com (accessed November 21, 2013).

12 Surrogacy in context

Ukraine and the United States

Delphine Lance & Jennifer Merchant

Introduction

The choice of these two countries is initially meant to highlight the fundamentally different legal/policy approaches that these states use, but also to point to contrasts in how surrogacy arrangements are carried out. This allows the authors to situate each "model" within its precise cultural and political environment, thus contributing to a more comprehensive knowledge of these different surrogacy processes.

Indeed, many countries – and even individual states in the US – have chosen to regulate surrogacy in a variety of ways. The different forms that these regulatory schemes take on naturally have an impact on the way citizens accept, integrate, or rebel against their constraints and even lack thereof.

The first part of this chapter will present the juridical and political framework governing surrogacy practices in these two countries. The second part will present fieldwork carried out in both countries, which will amply illustrate the context in which women who choose to engage in surrogacy in these two countries compose and interact with the legal superstructures that oversee their activities.

Juridical/Political frameworks governing surrogacy in Ukraine and the United States

Ukraine

Commercial surrogacy is legal in Ukraine; however, only for intended parents who are heterosexual married couples. Before beginning any aspect of an ART procedure, they must provide a marriage certificate to the agency or clinic. If the couple comes from another country, the marriage certificate must be in conformity with the October 5th 1961 La Hague Convention and notarised.[1]

According to Article 123 of the Ukrainian Family Code, intended parents are designated as such from the moment of conception.[2] It is illegal to declare the surrogate as the child's mother.[3] In a surrogacy case, it is the contract established between the surrogate and intended parents that allows for family ties, and not the delivery of the baby.

Article 319 of the Family Code stipulates that a woman registered as a child's mother can contest said established family ties. However, the surrogate cannot contest the genetic ties of the genetic mother and cannot keep the child at birth.

Additionally, surrogacy is only allowed under certain medical conditions: absence of uterus (genetic or due to hysterectomy); uterine cavity deformation; Asherman syndrome;[4] severe psychosomatic illness and/or symptoms rendering pregnancy impossible; or repeated failures (four at least) of embryo implantation in the uterus. Intentional parents must undergo a medical exam before the beginning of the procedure.

As for the surrogate, and in accordance with the *Directives on Reproductive Technology Procedures*,[5] she must already have a child who is mentally and physically healthy. If she is married, the Ukrainian Family Code does not call for the spouse's consent. Under the Ukrainian Family Law Code, spouses cannot intervene in each other's reproductive choices; however, agencies encourage intentional parents to obtain the consent of the husband for a very particular reason: Article 122 of the Ukrainian Family Code maintains the "presumption of paternity", in other words, the legal father is the man who is married to the woman who gives birth to a child. As such, the husband of the surrogate mother, if he so wishes, can contest the paternal family ties that the intended father wants established. Hence, it is necessary to obtain written consent from the husband of the surrogate.[6]

The *Directives* require the signature of a mutually consented contract between the intended parents and the surrogate before implantation of the embryo. If the intended parents are from abroad, the gestational surrogacy contract must be written in both Ukrainian and the language of the couple. It must indicate that the surrogate agrees to carry the child, that the child is not genetically related to her, and that at birth she will give the child to the couple. It must also stipulate that she relinquish her parental rights over the child. The future parents may add recommendations for the surrogate that may include nutritional advice and requests, the minimal number of visits to the doctor, etc.

It is important to bear in mind that the contract can evolve in the making and is not totally inflexible. As one lawyer explains:

> The contract is very extensive and the obligations of the surrogate mother as well ... everything is possible and each party carefully reads and then say "we would like to include this", and surrogate mother can respond "I do not like this clause", and we sit together and negotiate; it's not something that can't be changed, it's not fixed, it's up to the parties involved.

The contract also indicates that intended parents are fully responsible for the child at birth and must pay for all pregnancy expenses. According to Article 623 of the Ukrainian Civil Code, the amount of money that the surrogate receives must be negotiated between the couple and the surrogate. The average surrogacy contract is made up of two parts. The first part deals with the expenses and financial support of the surrogate. The couple must take on all expenses of the surrogate linked to the pregnancy throughout the entire procedure (medical costs, food, clothes, visits to the doctor, other trips, etc.). The second part of the contract directly concerns payment of the surrogate, a sum that is agreed upon from the start and cannot be modified afterwards.

The contract also anticipates any problems that may occur such as multiple births, the birth of a child afflicted with serious diseases or deformity, abortion for medical reasons, the divorce of the intended parents, etc. Also included in the agreement are any eventual sanctions to be levied against the surrogate in the event that she does not respect the contract, and which can range from a fine to the definitive cancellation of the contract.

Registering the child with the authorities is carried out by the intended parents. In fact, both their names are, from the start, recorded at the Family Registry Office. Requests for surrogates by foreign couples are handled in conformity with Ukrainian legislation. It is necessary to submit a certificate issued by a judge to the Family Registry Office that allows for the registration of the foreign couple as the legal parents of the child-to-be. The surrogate must also provide her written notary-approved consent. Her name appears in the column "Remarks". Only then may foreign couples apply for and obtain the birth certificate and passport of the child. This is only possible for foreigners whose own country recognises the legality of surrogacy procedures.

It is interesting to take note of a particular situation, that of a surrogacy arrangement carried out with anonymous donor gametes. In this case, the donor (sperm or egg) will never be able to obtain parental recognition or responsibility and/or rights over the child, and this in conformity with Paragraph 5.1 of the *Directives*. It is important to underline that in Ukraine, double-donation (sperm and egg) is prohibited in a surrogacy process. At least one of the intended parental couple's members must be genetically related to the child-to-be. And if there is a donation of egg or sperm, the donor's name is not mentioned in the contract at all.

In light of these different rules and regulations, some couples decide to proceed with a surrogacy arrangement without signing a contract. This can turn out to be a catastrophic situation. The couple can "abandon" the project at any time and leave the child to the surrogate, or on the contrary the surrogate can refuse to turn over the child.[7] In this case, the surrogate must take care of the child she did not want from the start, or the parents must give up hope of retrieving their child or else initiate litigation in the hopes that a judge will rule in their favour.

A few remarks, in conclusion, concerning the child's nationality when her/his parents are foreign: under Ukrainian citizenship law, no mention is made of the fact that a child born of a surrogate mother is automatically Ukrainian. S/he will in fact obtain the nationality of her/his parents. S/he will only be automatically Ukrainian if her/his parents are permanent residents of the Ukraine or if s/he cannot obtain the foreign nationality of the parents. If s/he obtains her/his parents' nationality, the Ukrainian regime governing foreigners is applied. Indeed, the Ukraine has concluded a great number of international agreements with many countries, thus allowing foreigners to stay at least three months in the Ukraine without a visa.

The United States

In the United States, recourse to ART falls under federal jurisprudence that situates these acts within the realm of the private sphere, one supported by the existence of a constitutional "right to privacy" reiterated in several US Supreme Court decisions in the realm of non-procreation.[8] In addition, the US Supreme Court declared in 1998 that procreation was a "major life activity" protected by the Americans with Disabilities Act.[9] Recourse to ART is then more or less regulated by different public policy approaches throughout the 50 states.

Contrary to what is generally assumed, ART practices do not evolve in a "no man's land". Despite the extensive constitutional protection of private procreative choices guaranteed by the aforementioned decisions, this does not mean that a US citizen can do anything s/he wants when seeking ART (Merchant, 2010).

First of all, one must quote the existence of two federal laws that govern ART practices:

- The National Organ Transplant Act[10] prohibits the sale of organs and other elements of the human body (hence what has a commercial value in sperm and egg donation is the time sacrificed, salaries lost and eventual dangers incurred by the donors).
- The second national law requires the Health and Human Services Department to publish an annual activity report of all the infertility treatment centres and clinics in operation across the country.[11] In 2012, 456 clinics out of the 483 clinics responded. No sanctions are provided in the event that a clinic does not respond, apart from the one inflicted by potential patients who systematically consult the report before choosing a clinic.

The absence of any other type of national ART legislation is quite simply explained by the principle of the separation of powers and the functioning of US federalism. Article 1 Section 8 of the US Constitution attributes to Congress a certain number of explicit (reserved) powers and obligations. The remaining implicit (unmentioned) powers are attributed to the states and the people in virtue of the Ninth and Tenth Amendments to the Constitution. From a practical standpoint, this simply means that the states and their institutions – their representative assemblies, their courts – have the power to create and implement public policy in a wide range of activities: healthcare policy, family law policy, education, penal law, etc. In the realm of ART, many states have laws or rely on common law precedents, some more restrictive than others, like Louisiana; some more liberal than others, like California.

First and foremost, it is important to underline the fact that surrogacy is not frequent. There are approximately four million births per year in the United States, and among them around 1,000 to 1,500 births through surrogacy; in other words, about 1% of all ART practices. In addition, half of these births are for foreign couples.[12] These figures have remained constant since the Centers for Disease Control and Prevention (CDC) has been publishing its annual reports, from 1998.

It is also erroneous to assume that most surrogacy arrangements end up before the courts. According to the American Bar Association, litigation due to conflict in surrogacy agreements/contracts is situated at approximately 0.1% of all surrogacy procedures, in other words, around two cases per year go before the courts.

On the other hand, it is possible to criticise the lack of coherence in laws governing surrogacy: who has access, who can be a surrogate, the different and uneven modalities for establishing family ties, the important differences in payment for surrogates, etc. This creates a complex national panorama that de facto installs an inequality among women who become surrogates and a complicated and oftentimes confusing situation for couples seeking a surrogate in all legality.

Many voices are increasingly being heard in the US calling for the need to withdraw surrogacy agreements from the realm of private contract law and place them within the framework of public health and/or public law practices. Two attempts at this on the federal level were initiated in the early 1990s, as well as two other bills simply calling for the abolition of surrogacy altogether, to no avail.

Hence, we still face a decentralised and piecemeal approach to the issue, one that plays out more or less as follows:

- Four states do not recognise any form whatsoever of a surrogacy agreement or contract.
- Four states recognise the validity of a surrogacy contract but with no monetary exchange whatsoever, i.e. altruistic surrogacy.
- Four states recognise the validity of a surrogacy contract with payment.
- Three states recognise the validity of a surrogacy contract with payment but not exceeding medical costs, clothing, loss of salary of the surrogate once she goes on maternity leave, and other attending costs. These states also accept by law that a surrogate may breach the contract after birth and keep the child.
- Seven states totally prohibit surrogacy, and criminalise it.
- All the other states have no law governing surrogacy, leaving these arrangements up to private law contracts, and in the event of litigation, the courts step in.

Some examples of surrogacy regulation

Ten states that authorise surrogacy arrangements have very detailed laws governing these practices. Four of them – Florida, Utah, Washington and New Hampshire – present what corresponds, to many analysts, to a public health approach to framing surrogacy practices. All four states require by law most if not all of the following criteria:

1 The intended parents must be at least 21 years of age and residents of the state for at least one year.
2 They must submit to thorough physical and psychological exams, as well as to a home study (as occurs in the case of adoption).
3 The intended mother must prove that she is incapable of carrying a child.

4   At least one of the intended parents must be genetically related to the child-to-be.

5   The surrogate must also be at least 21 years of age and resident of the state for at least one year.

6   She must already have a healthy child. Her eggs may not be used in the process.

7   She also must submit to thorough physical and psychological exams, and a home study.

8   She must not be a beneficiary of any form of social welfare (food stamps, Medicaid).

9   Payment must not exceed medical costs, clothing, days/salary lost due to illness and or maternity leave, and all other legal costs.

10 Both parties must have their own lawyers, and the contract negotiated and written up before the ART procedure of implantation must be approved by a judge.

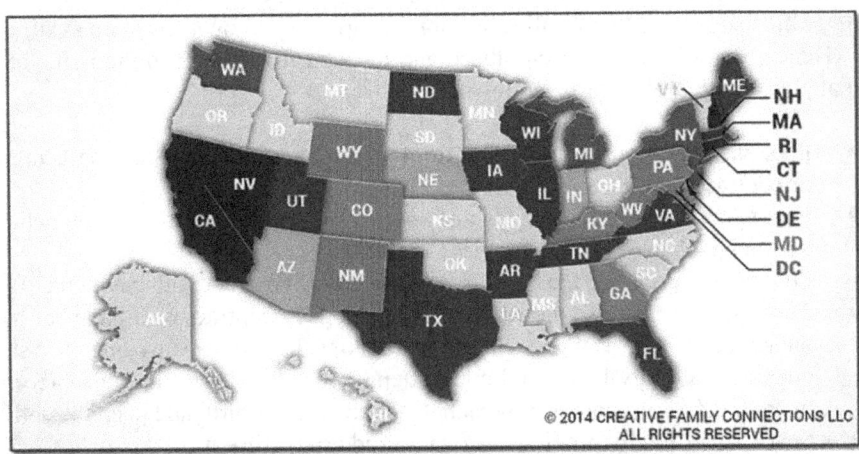

CLICK ON A STATE ABOVE FOR INFORMATION ON STATE LAWS

GREEN LIGHT STATES

● **Green Without Conditions:** Statute or case law supports or reliable result

CA, CT, DE, NH, NV, RI*

● **Green With Conditions:** Statute Or Case Law Permits If Certain Conditions Are Met (Eg, May Be Restrictions For Marital Status, Sexual Orientation, Genetic Tie To Child) Or Post-Birth Parentage Order Granted Only

AR, FL, IA, IL, MA, ME, ND, TN, TX, UT, VA*, WI

● **Statute Or Case Law Permits But Uncertainty Remains Or Results Vary By Venue**

MD, NM, PA, WY, WV

VACUUM STATES - Surrogacy Permitted Because No Statute or Case Law Prohibits

● **Pre-Birth Parentage Order Granted In Most Cases**

CO, GA, KY

● **Parentage Order Granted If Certain Conditions Are Met (Eg, There May Be Restrictions For Marital Status, Sexual Orientation, Genetic Tie To Child) Or Post-Birth Order Only**

AK, AL, HI, ID, KS, LA, MN, MO, MS, MT, NC, OH, OK, OR, SC, SD, VT

OTHER STATES

● **Yellow Light:** Caution, Proceed With Extreme Caution! Statue Makes Surrogacy Contracts Unenforceable, but Some Courts Grant Parentage Orders

AZ, IN, NE*

● **Red Light:** Statute Or Case Law Prohibits Surrogacy Contracts

DC, MI, NJ, NY, WA

Figure 12.1 Gestational surrogacy across the United States: state-by-state map for commercial surrogacy

www.creativefamilyconnections.com/#!surrogacy-law-by-state/f49jq

Social and cultural realities in the United States and Ukraine

Let us now turn to the means and way surrogacy is represented and experienced by women who choose to be surrogates in both countries. This contextualisation will allow the reader to better understand what surrogates experience and the way they represent this procedure that they embark upon. As such, the reader will observe that it is not because surrogacy is legal that it is accepted or considered acceptable. Its practice can be the source of controversy and reprobation even though it is legal. Likewise it is not because surrogacy is illegal that it is not practised.

Hence, the reader will be able to better observe how women define their practice in function of specific socio-cultural contexts, and how they compose and interact with normative structures, by which we mean more specifically ethical, religious and family frameworks.

This will lead us to discuss the manner in which these women represent their "journey", their role, and how they perceive their body during the surrogacy process. This in turn will allow us to better understand the "agency" these women exercise and allow us to question the notion of "ethical surrogacy". Last but not least, we will be able to better understand how surrogates negotiate with the cultural, moral and ethical elements present in their personal lives as well as those of the society they live in.

From the standpoint of the French bioethics debate

One way of beginning this analysis is to use the political, social and ethical discourse in France surrounding the practice of surrogacy as a benchmark. The main question that is raised is whether or not an ethical form of surrogacy is possible, and if so, what are the required elements that contribute to making it ethical? It is common among French intellectuals, associations (e.g. Le Corp) and public authorities (e.g. Comité Consultatif National d'Ethique – CCNE) to either denounce any and all forms of surrogacy, or to oppose what is perceived as an ethical form of surrogacy, carried out in the United States, to an unethical form, carried out in Ukraine or India (Busnel et al., 2009; Agacinski, 2009; Thery, 2014). In previous fieldwork of same-sex couples and their recourse to surrogacy abroad, Delphine Lance found that this discursive opposition, highly present in France, allowed these couples, and in some cases almost forced them, to adopt the comparison between an "unethical" Ukrainian context and an "ethical" North American one. In short, surrogates were exploited in Ukraine because they were poor and not in the United States because they were not poor (see also Ragoné, 1994). For these persons and other associations interviewed during previous fieldwork, it became crucial to construct an ideal ethical surrogacy model, which came to be defined as follows:

> For us, we can only accept what we call 'ethical surrogacy' practices wherein all actors – the surrogate, the intended parents, and last but not least, the child to be – are taken into account and listened to, and that their fundamental rights and personal identities be respected and accompanied throughout the

procedure. 'Ethical surrogacy', far from being the horrific context many point to by relying on some of the most extreme examples of abuse, can be one of the most beautiful human experiences of all, one that is highly respectful and profoundly inspired by values promoting the equality of the sexes, and the dignity and rights of women and children.[13]

In one interview, the President of a same-sex family rights association argued that, indeed, surrogacy was exploitative in Ukraine because the procedures did not respect the surrogate's dignity, incited people to commit fraud, and did not strive for the building of a relationship both present and future with the surrogate, the ensuing child, and the intended parents, this being the ultimate guarantee of ethical conduct in a surrogacy process. It is interesting to note that these are the same arguments pronounced by the most fervent French opponents to any form of surrogacy (Agacinski, 2009).

Hence, there are two types of surrogacy for those persons and members of this association in favour of surrogacy: one that is non-ethical because it is alienating (Frydman and Eliacheff, 2008), commodifies the body, is indignant, and usually is practised in "Southern" and "Eastern" countries, notably India and Ukraine; and one that is ethical, transparent, and above all "altruistic", more commonly practiced and found in "Northern" countries. A hierarchy is thus clearly established, and we are in the presence of what one analyst has called the "West and the Rest" (Sahlins, 1976).

It is out of the transnational reality of surrogacy practices and this hierarchisation of models that present-day fieldwork, which will now be presented, was launched. Indeed, it had become obvious that a comparison was in order and could enhance our understanding of these practices, if only through the actual presentation of how they transpire in both areas of the world. In any event, the comparison would strive, at least in part, to reveal exactly how the process unfolds beyond any preconceptions and/or "speculations" pronounced beforehand (Pande, 2010).

Once the choice was made to start from the opposition constructed in French bioethics debates over surrogacy, certain important questions emerged. What was more pertinent, to compare countries or practices? Wasn't it above all important to realise that we are at present caught up in different economic and social realities that do not allow us to analyse from a "Eurocentric" perspective (Pande, 2010)? Isn't it also important to integrate into our analyses the concept of women's empowerment? Faced with these questions, we opted for a pluralist approach to the processes observed in both Ukraine and the United States, in an effort to minimise the direct opposition of both countries and, rather, to study each of them through the prism of the other, and above all to focus on the practices established in each country.

Surrogates in Ukraine

Fieldwork that will now be presented is based on more than eight months spent in Ukraine and five months in the United States, during which more than 60 interviews were carried out with Ukrainian and American surrogates.

Insofar as Ukraine is concerned, 33 interviews were carried out with surrogates who were between the ages of 19 and 34 and all mothers of at least one child. More than half of them were divorced and lived, for the majority of them, with their family (parents and/or grandparents). Their educational level was quite heterogeneous, ranging from a junior high school diploma (around 15 years old) to a university Master's degree. More than half of these women worked – professor, banker, factory worker – or were on maternity leave.

Some of these Ukrainian women were relieved to be able to speak with someone about their experience, and even found it positive that socio-anthropological work was being done on the topic. That being said, it was absolutely necessary for them that their anonymity be preserved. A few among them seemed *a priori* reluctant to speak of their experiences, but in the end agreed to do so once they were assured that they would remain anonymous. It was indeed very important for some of these women not to mention the town or city they came from, because even if their close family members knew what they were doing, they did not want their surroundings and neighbours to know. Indeed, even though surrogacy is legal in Ukraine, it is not socially acceptable. The majority of Ukrainian women encountered moved away from their hometown at around six months gestation to a smaller individual apartment, far from their region and close to the clinic they were working with, where they could also invite their own families to visit.

Lance carried out an informal poll on surrogacy in general among 50 Ukrainians.[14] Most of them had no idea that surrogacy was practised in their country. Only five persons out of 50 considered surrogacy as positive and deemed altruistic. Most of the others equated surrogacy to baby-selling and considered it totally immoral. This expression of immorality is based on religious beliefs and practices (Greco-Catholic or Orthodox) or on certain gendered stereotypes that assimilate a woman to the loving mother incapable of "selling" her baby. Olga, a PhD student in ethics, said, "To be honest, I don't understand their choices; there are jobs in Ukraine. Why are they doing it? Why do these women exploit the poor parents who have infertility problems – that's horrible."

In this case, one may thus observe that the surrogate is designated as being responsible for the exploitation perceived of in a surrogacy process, contrary to more classical feminist positions that see these practices as being exploitive of the surrogate's body (Corea, 1985; Raymond, 1994). Within this framework, it appears to be more pertinent to explore, as Rudrappa and Forest (2014) do in the Indian context, the reasons why certain women, despite social disapproval, decide nonetheless to engage in a surrogacy process. In the case of Ukraine, one must turn to financial motivations that serve as the basic reason.

Fieldwork then brought Lance to spend five months in the United States, where she carried out 27 interviews with surrogates aged 26 to 43 years of age, and who all had at least one child. All but one, who was divorced, were either married or living with a partner. Their educational level ranged from high school diploma to university Master's degree. They were from and evolved within a middle-class socio-economic category.

Contrary to Ukraine, surrogacy is socially acceptable in the United States (Ragoné, 1994), and Lance never encountered persons who expressed hostility to surrogacy in general or to her work.

The first theme studied flows directly from the French contention of more or less alienating and exploitative surrogacy procedures according to the country examined. The second theme involves the religious dimension of surrogacy. This aspect quickly emerged as a very interesting and important one to analyse as it serves as a privileged vector in the manner to perceive of, within a given cultural context, surrogacy practices, and highlights the way women act in function of the context they evolve in.

Thinking "gift" and "money" at the same time

> How can one accept that an impoverished woman carry our child ? This is not ethical (…) Our surrogate told us, it is a gift she is giving us, money doesn't have that much importance.
>
> (Benjamin, father in surrogacy process in the US)

> I say to myself that thanks to the money we give her, she will be able to improve her standard of living, so in that sense it is not a negative thing.
>
> (Paul, father in surrogacy process in Ukraine)

Two persons, two countries, and radically opposed discourses on surrogacy and money. But how is the "money question" dealt with by the surrogates? Is the fact that some women choose to engage in a surrogacy process just for money a legitimate enough reason to condemn these practices, as do those who are against surrogacy or only for "ethical" surrogacy? From our standpoint, the act of opposing surrogate motivations between countries does not suffice to allow us to conclude as to what is ethical and what is not.

Indeed, previous empirical studies demonstrate the absence of pertinence in transposing discursive logics relative to surrogacy practices from one country to another. While the rhetoric of a "gift of life" in the United States (Ragoné, 1994) or a "gift as a relation" (Teman, 2010) in Israel serve as predominant motivations for surrogates in their engagement, these cannot be compared to the logic present in so-called "Southern" countries. Pande would explain, for example, that the "gift-giving metaphor does not work when class difference and structural inequality between the potential gift giver and gift taker is so large" (Pande, 2011: 7).

Economic differences between surrogates and intended parents render the "altruistic gift" metaphor obsolete, and surrogates in this context prefer to use the rhetoric of the "gift of God". As for the anthropologists Sayantan DasGupta and Shamita Das Dasgupta, they give cultural reasons for differences in perception of the gift. According to them, "gift-giving" does not mean much in Indian society, where emphasis is placed more on "value relationships over autonomy, interdependence over self-governance and group identity over individualism" (DasGupta and Dasgupta, 2010: 140). These are important points raised by ethnographers and highlight the indispensable importance of empirical comparisons.

The financial motivation to become a surrogate

In Ukraine, the average salary is 3,509 grivnas per month (approximately 300 euros per month at the time of the fieldwork). Therefore, certain women think that surrogacy could solve their financial problems and/or improve their standard of living. In this framework, surrogacy can appear to be a sort of "survival strategy" (Pande, 2010: 972), such as in the case of Oksana (33 years of age, a surrogate for a Russian couple):

> I've been surrogate mother once, just because I really needed a big amount of money, more than 100,000 hrn [approximately 10,000 euros at the time of the fieldwork]. Debts are needed to be paid, I have two kids. No way out.

Oksana spoke to us about surrogacy in quasi-military terms. She compared male military service duty in her country to female reproductive labour. The majority of women encountered in Ukraine justified their decision to become a surrogate in terms of duty to their family. Thus, thanks to surrogacy, these women expressed satisfaction in being able to contribute financially to support their families (sometimes up to three generations live under one roof). This vision of the woman as being automatically or "naturally" altruistic is predominant in the Ukraine. From what is generally frowned upon socially, some women were/are able to negotiate the transition to a socially acceptable image of themselves as surrogates based on cultural assumptions of what a woman is, and thus put forth the fact that they are helping their families, which in turn can valorise their role as a surrogate.

Concerning financial motivations, a certain number of other women decide to engage in a surrogacy process with the objective of emancipating themselves or obtaining a higher social rank. In this case, surrogacy can be seen as a form of "empowerment" (Rudrappa and Forest, 2014). Because of surrogacy, these women are able to buy an apartment and live independently from their parents/extended family. They can also go back to school or university, or start a new professional training program. Lena, 20 years old and mother of a four-year-old, was able to start medical school after being a surrogate. She explained that being a surrogate made it possible for her to avoid being an employee for five years before going to medical school. Even though her relatives and surroundings frown upon surrogacy, she explained that because of surrogacy she was able to protect herself and her child in the "long term" and guarantee their future. Tiffany, previously an American surrogate for friends of hers, renewed the experience with the objective of then opening up her own surrogacy agency, as she needed the down payment for such a business venture. In this instance, she used her own experience as a surrogate to valorise her decision to open her own agency, rendering it all the more legitimate. In these situations, money earned through surrogacy allowed these women to enjoy a degree of autonomy they might not have found elsewhere.

A certain number of other women perceive of being a surrogate as a far more attractive option than other types of jobs. Lioudmila said:

> He [Husband] wasn't supportive from the beginning, he said there can be consequences. But I said if I go to factory for work, to the leather factory and if I breathe glue, I will spoil my health in one year, but in other case I have a chance to help people.

Surrogacy from this perspective is seen as an enlargement of one's possible options (Guillarme, 2003), and has an added value in light of the fact that the surrogate is helping a couple achieve their dream of having a child.

Surrogacy as alienating?

The vast majority of surrogates perceive of what they are doing as a job, or, like Tiffany, make it into one. Certain feminists criticise this vision of gestation as being a form of employment. In her criticism of the political theory of the contract, Carole Pateman (2010) pronounces herself against surrogacy contracts. According to her, these amount to a new way of oppressing women. The alienation brought on by the surrogacy contract is all the more evident in that it involves the total body of the woman at all times and for nine months. She writes:

> Her personhood is at stake in the deepest sense of the word. She relinquishes her physiological, emotional and uniquely creative rights of her body, in other words, her rights as a woman. For nine months, she enters into the most intimate relationship there is with a developing human being who is a part of her.
>
> (Pateman, 2010: 296)

Deborah Satz criticises this approach, which she sees as being far too essentialist, since nothing can justify the procreative act as being more a part of one's identity than her/his relationships with friends and family. The majority of Ukrainian and American surrogates encountered explain that they were able to separate their "selves" from the gestational process and thus avoid any sense of "alienation". The use of self-qualifying words such as "baby-sitter", "chicken", and, more commonly, "oven" and/or "incubator/инкубатор", allowed them to measure their degree of emotional attachment. The term "incubator", used by both Ukrainian and American surrogates, did not reduce them to simple "mother machines (Corea, 1985), for all those interviewed consider the artificial uterus as "inhuman" because it is detached from any kind of human relationship.

This puzzle-like approach to the body, as Elly Teman (2010) has demonstrated in her impressive concept of "body-map", allows these women to preserve themselves. This method of compartmentalising things allows them to attribute corporal sensations to diverse emotions that sometimes do and sometimes don't create ties. This fragmentation thus allows them to avoid experiencing a sense of alienation since, by symbolically dividing up their body into specific portions, their self is preserved as it is distinct from their womb. Hence one may speak of what Charis Thompson calls "agency through objectification" (Thompson, 2007).

Exploitation?

For the majority of the Ukrainian women interviewed, they do not perceive of themselves as being exploited. They speak more of a process that they perceive of as a "win–win" situation (Rozée and Unisa, 2014). The rhetoric around money and financial assistance is thus more easily used to motivate the decision to become a surrogate. These two dimensions – helping others and being paid – are not incompatible and do not cancel each other out. The rhetoric of "gift" in these cases is valorised by a certain idea present in Mauss' gift/counter-gift paradigm (Mauss, 1968). Jessica, a 23-year-old surrogate, says: "If you can help someone and someone can help you, I think it's good."

The majority of the Ukrainian women Lance encountered did not work with agencies or other types of brokers, hence they were the ones who "fixed the price". One may thus question whether the very concept of exploitation is pertinent since the price fixed by the surrogate is deemed just and equitable by herself (Macklin, 2014). The problem of exploitation is a very interesting and important one encountered during fieldwork. When some Ukrainian surrogates Lance interviewed learnt of the amount of money American surrogates receive – approximately 25,000 US dollars – and they compared that to what they earned and their standard of living, they expressed dismay as to why agency surrogates don't organise and rebel against what the Ukrainian agencies seemingly do, that is, underpay their surrogates.

As for American surrogates, they point to Ukraine and India and decry what they see as perfect examples of how surrogates there are exploited because they are poor and only do it for money. It is looking through these lenses that the analyst realises how essential it is to take into consideration the social and cultural system wherein surrogacy practices are being carried out. Along this vein, the question of religion emerges, acting like a magnifying glass to demonstrate to what extent analysing surrogacy, especially in terms of ethics, cannot deprive itself of social and cultural constructions.

The role of religion in the surrogacy process

In France, apart from the aforementioned ethical debate, one may also find another arena of tense debate, i.e. surrounding the position of the Catholic church on surrogacy, a practice that it considers as contrary to the rights of the child. A totally different religious approach to surrogacy is found in the United States.

Gayle, for example, said:

> I am a Christian and wanted to make sure that it wasn't something that I shouldn't do for somebody else and so we actually went to the church and talked with the Pastor about me being a surrogate mother to make sure there wasn't any reason in the Bible why I shouldn't be. Our Pastor instructed us

that Mary was in fact a surrogate mother and she carried Jesus and obviously Jesus was God's child so I really felt confident after talking with him that everything would be fine and there wasn't anything wrong with me doing that, scripturally from a Biblical standpoint. So much of the time the Church teaches you to give to the orphans and take care of the widows and those that are hungry, to feed them, and I think from a Biblical standpoint, it teaches us to give without necessarily receiving in return.

Hence, we are in the presence of a different interpretation of the Bible than the one put forth by the Catholic Church in France, which does not think of Mary as the surrogate mother of Jesus. Yet, from the interpretation that Gayle's Pastor gives, surrogacy becomes possible, even applauded. Lance spent several days with Gayle and also met the Pastor and interviewed him. His position was straightforward: God allows us to bring forth children thanks to new reproductive technologies; why refuse this progress?

The Ukrainian situation is quite interesting as it is somewhat a blended and condensed version of both the US and French contexts. The Orthodox Church in East Ukraine, where the majority of interviews were carried out, is the main religious institution in this region. However, there is not a consensus within this church on the position to take relative to surrogacy. Indeed, each parish organises itself as it wishes, in an independent manner. Consequently, from one parish to the next, diverging positions on surrogacy can be found. This heterogeneity was what prompted and subsequently allowed Oksana to harmonise her religious beliefs and her church with her decision to become a surrogate. She explains:

> I've been to a church and asked about it. At one of the churches, I was told that it's not good. But in another one, I was told that the church accepts this (surrogacy) because you don't sleep with another man, it is made by medicine. In fact Virgin Mary, how did she give birth? So this way they think it is normal.

Indeed, Oksana felt she needed church benediction to proceed with being a surrogate, decided not to remain passive, and set out to find the place where she would receive this benediction. She found it in the approval of a priest, free as they are to interpret the situation, just as the Ukrainian women are free to change churches/priests so they may feel spiritually in accordance with the decision to go ahead with being a surrogate.

Conclusion

This brief comparative study is not meant to present US and Ukrainian surrogacy motivations as being analogous. Rather, it is meant to allow the reader to perceive of the manner in which each woman, in function of framework and structures she is set within, thinks of and carries out a surrogacy engagement.

Indeed, as this text demonstrates, there are various political, social, and cultural contexts from which surrogacy practices emerge, and which led either quickly or not to some sort of public policy regulation or none at all. The different forms of regulation that one may observe in Ukraine or in the United States obviously then have an impact on how surrogacy actors and agents engage in the process, even when prohibited. These different negotiations make up what is interesting, for it is through their analysis that one may understand the multiple ways in which women who choose to become surrogates deal with the process.

In short, there is not on the one hand women who are exploited and on the other hand women who are free; this dualism is far too simple a prism for the complex social phenomenon that is surrogacy. What one can tentatively conclude is that there are women who, according to their life experiences and the structures they depend on, engage in surrogacy procedures, all the while attempting to remain the main actors/agents of the experience as a whole.

Notes

1 The Hague Convention, 1961, rendering obsolete the requirement that foreign public acts be legalised.
2 Family Law Code, re-issued in 2004.
3 Certain Ukrainian agencies do so nonetheless.
4 Uterine affliction provoking the absence of monthly periods.
5 *Directives on Reproductive Technology Procedures,* Ukrainian Health Ministry Order, No. 771, 12/23/2008.
6 Even though this is not required, all agencies studied insisted on having the surrogate husband's written consent.
7 In Ukraine, the first hypothesis is the most observed.
8 *Skinner vs State of Oklahoma, ex. rel. Williamson,* 316 U.S. 535 (1942), *Griswold vs Connecticut,* 381 U.S. 479 (1965), *Roe vs Wade, 410 U.S. 113* (1973). For further reference, see Merchant, 2006.
9 *Bragdon vs Abbott,* 524 U.S. 624 (1998).
10 The National Organ Transplant Act (Pub. L. 98–507), 1984.
11 The Fertility Clinic Success Rate and Certification Act (FCSRCA) of 1992 mandates that clinics performing ART annually provide data for all procedures performed to CDC. CDC is required to use these data to report and publish clinic-specific success rates. The first report, the *1995 Assisted Reproductive Technology Success Rates Report,* was released in December 1997. Here is the link to the latest report of 2012: http://www.cdc.gov/art/reports/2012/national-summary.html
12 http://www.cdc.gov/art/pdf/2012-report/national-summary/art_2012_national_summary_report.pdf
13 Silberfeld, J., 2011, Alexandre Urwicz: "Aujourd'hui, nous ne défendons plus notre gaytitude mais nos familles", available from http://yagg.com/2011/03/03/alexandre-urwicz-aujourdhui-nous-ne-defendons-plus-notre-gaytitude-mais-nos-familles/
14 Between October 2012 and May 2013, with 50 Ukrainians from Lviv and Kiev.

References

Agacinski S., *Corps en miettes*, Paris: Flammarion, 2009.
Busnel M.C., Frydman R., Szejer M.,Winter J.P., *Abandon sur ordonnance, manifeste contre la légalisation des mères porteuses*, Paris: Bayard, 2009.
Corea G., *The Mother Machine: Reproductive Technologies from Artificial Insemination to Artificial Wombs*, New York: Harper and Row, 1985.

DasGupta S., Dasgupta S. D., Motherhood Jeopardized: Reproductive Technologies in Indian Communities. In Wendy Chavkin and Jane Maree Maher (eds), *The Globalization of Motherhood: Deconstructions and Reconstructions of Biology and Care*, New York: Routledge, pp. 131–153, 2010.

Frydman R., Eliacheff C., Mère porteuse, à quel prix? *Le Monde*, 30 Janvier, 2008.

Guillarme B., Louer son ventre, *Raisons politiques*, 4(12) :77–83, 2003.

Macklin R., *Don, contre-don et rémunération des gamètes dans l'assistance médicale à la procréation*, Séminaire, Conférence organisée par Jennifer Merchant et Laurence Brunet, Paris Sorbonne, Novembre 2014.

Mauss M., Essai sur le don: Forme et raison de l'échange dans les sociétés archaïques, in *Sociologie et anthropologie PUF, Collection Quadrige, 4th edn*, 1968.

Merchant J., *Procréation et politique aux Etats-Unis: 1965–2005*, Paris: Belin, 2006.

Merchant J., Assisted Reproductive Technology (ART) in the United States: Towards a National Regulatory Framework?, *International Journal of Bioethics*, 20(4):3–4, 2010.

Pande A., Commercial Surrogacy in India: Manufacturing a Perfect Mother Worker, *Signs: Journal of Women in Culture and Society*, (35)4:969–992, 2010.

Pande A., Transnational commercial surrogacy in India: gifts for global sisters? *Reproductive BioMedicine Online*, 23:618–662, 2011.

Pateman C., *Le contrat sexuel* (1988), Paris: La Découverte, 2010.

Ragoné H., *Surrogate Motherhood: Conception in the Heart*, Boulder: Westview Press, 1994.

Raymond J., *Women as Wombs: Reproductive Technologies and the Battle Over Women's Freedom*, Melbourne, Australia: Spinifex Press, 1994.

Rozée V., Unisa S., Surrogacy from a reproductive rights perspective: the case of India, *Autrepart*, 70:185–203, 2014.

Rudrappa S., Forest M., Des ateliers de confection aux lignes d'assemblage des bébés: Stratégies d'emploi parmi des mères porteuses à Bangalore, Inde, *Cahier du genre*, 56:59–86, 2014.

Sahlins M., *Culture and Practical Reason*, Chicago: University of Chicago Press, 1976.

Satz D., Markets in Women's Reproductive Labor, *Philosophy and Public Affairs*, 21(2), 1992.

Teman E., *Birthing a Mother: The Surrogate Body and the Pregnant Self*, Berkeley: University of California Press, 2010.

Thery I., GPA: pour un débat argumenté et respectueux des personnes, *Libération*, 23 Juillet 2014.

Thompson C., *Making Parents: The Ontological Choreography of Reproductive Technologies*, Cambridge, Massachusetts: MIT Press, 2007.

13 Local surrogacy in a global circuit

The embodied intimacies of Israeli surrogacy arrangements

Elly Teman

Introduction

Today the word *surrogacy* seems to go hand in hand with the notion of "cross-border reproductive tourism," and much of the scholarly discussion of surrogacy is dominated by a focus on global concerns about this practice. At the center of cross-border surrogacy is the understanding that individuals entering these arrangements are often from different nationalities, frequently do not speak the same language and hold diverse cultural understandings about money, kinship and technology (Pande 2011; Deomampo 2013; Vora 2014). These cross-border arrangements have also been critiqued for the inequalities of race and class that they perpetuate through arrangements in which dominant classes from the West rely on the reproductive labor of women of low economic status in developing nations (Harrison 2014).

Within this global and cross-border framework, the case of surrogacy in Israel emerges as a very particular, local and nationally bounded case in which surrogacy arrangements take place in a starkly different context than that emergent on the global circuit. Whereas surrogacy arrangements in the developing world often take place in uncertain regulatory frameworks, Israel's surrogacy law of 1996 not only legalized the practice but also regulates and monitors it closely. The law sanctioned a state-appointed committee to supervise all surrogacy agreements that take place on Israeli soil and any arrangements that do not receive the committee's approval are criminalized (Teman 2010a; 2010b).

The law also specifically eliminates the possibility of cross-border, international and even inter-religious surrogacy arrangements on Israeli soil. Only Israeli citizens and permanent residents are eligible to enter into these contracts, and the state committee restrictively screens all applicants' criminal backgrounds, psychological competence and medical health before allowing them to proceed. The surrogacy law prohibits "traditional surrogacy" in which the surrogate is the genetic mother of the baby, instead allowing only gestational surrogacy, which is dependent on IVF technology. All arrangements must be medically assisted by state-approved clinics that are subject to close government regulation.

In order to gain the committee's approval, the intended mother must establish medical documents proving she does not have a uterus, that her life is endangered by pregnancy, or that she has undergone at least eight failed attempts to become pregnant through IVF or had at least seven miscarriages. Thus, unlike the marketing of surrogacy in India to foreign couples as a commercial, economically lucrative offshoot of medical tourism and "outsourcing" with limited state interference (Harrison 2014), the Israeli surrogacy law aims to keep surrogacy an extremely limited, local, national, practice.

This local practice is even more particular in that it is aimed at producing religiously legitimate Jewish citizens. The law was significantly influenced by state officials who wished to keep surrogacy as "kosher" as possible in terms of Jewish law and thus ensure the acceptability of surrogacy among a wide range of rabbis (Kahn 2000; Teman 2010b). Because many rabbis interpret the religion of the child as determined by the religion of the birth mother, the surrogate must be of the same religious denomination as both intended parents; the committee will consider an inter-religious agreement only if all the parties are not Jewish. Moreover, since in Jewish law a child born by a married surrogate to a married man who is not her husband could be considered the product of adulterous relations, the surrogacy law originally required all surrogates to be single, widowed or divorced.[1] And since some rabbis may consider a surrogate carrying an embryo created from her brother's sperm as incest, the surrogacy law does not allow any genetic relation between surrogate and intended parents.

As a result of this very restricted pool of participants in local surrogacy arrangements in Israel, the women who participated in my long-term (1998–2006) ethnographic study of Israeli surrogacy arrangements shared a very specific set of characteristics (Teman 2010a).[2] All of the surrogates and intended mothers were Jewish-Israeli citizens. Surrogates were single or divorced, raising at least one child of their own, and couples hiring surrogates were married or legally, heterosexually paired, because the law prohibits same-sex couples and single persons from hiring surrogates. Surrogates motivations were primarily financial, but most were not desperately poor. Most couples were Israeli middle class and able to afford surrogacy only because all medical aspects, including unlimited (and otherwise prohibitively expensive) embryo transfers, were heavily subsidized through Israel's social medicine system. Most of the couples financed the surrogate's fee and other expenses by way of loans, selling their car, or mortgaging their house.

Since Israel is such a tiny country, participants interacted far more frequently and intensely than what might be possible in transnational surrogacies and even in US surrogacies, where surrogates and couples usually live in different states. While many of the clinics in India prevent surrogates and intended parents from ever meeting one another, or restrict their interaction to one or two supervised meetings (Harrison 2014), all of the surrogates and intended parents in my study had not only met but routinely interacted with one another without mediation throughout the process. In contrast to cross-border Indian surrogacy arrangements in which spoken language barriers and surrogate illiteracy mean that any communication between the parties involved usually necessitates an interpreter (Deomampo 2013), the women in my study all shared the common spoken and written language of Hebrew.

Participants also shared cultural knowledge, including basic cultural attitudes and understandings toward motherhood and childbearing. Surrogates and intended mothers alike had been socialized into a cultural realm often characterized as "obsessed" with motherhood and fertility (Kahn 2000), where "non-natalist" voices are seldom heard in public and private arenas, even as being "childfree by choice" has become a legitimate social option in many other societies (Donath 2010). Intended mothers all agreed that they would do anything to have a child, and some had gone through up to 30 IVF attempts before turning to surrogacy. Surrogacy was viewed as a "last resort" before adoption and a process through which they hoped to participate in the pregnancy rather than "receive a baby through the mail," as one interviewee referred to adoption.

In line with this cultural attitude toward childbearing, surrogates did not usually encounter stigmatic or critical attitudes regarding their role from their families and friends. Unlike Indian surrogates, who sometimes hide their pregnancies by moving away from home for the duration of their surrogacy to avoid accusations of prostitution or infidelity (Pande 2011), the Israeli surrogates largely took pride in their role and shared it with everyone they knew. There was no question in their eyes that what they were doing – making another woman into a mother – was just about the biggest *mitzvah*, or good deed, a woman could do. And they seemed to inherently understand the intended mothers' desire to be part of the process; nearly all of the surrogates encouraged the intended mother to participate in the pregnancy as much as possible.

In the following, I argue that it is because of the restricted nature of these arrangements within this nationally, culturally and geographically bounded space that the type of surrogacy emergent in Israel creates a starkly different narrative than that emergent from the transnational Indian context. I argue that within this local practice of surrogacy it is intimacy and sameness, rather than distance and otherness, which emerge as key frames of the surrogacy arrangement.

Specifically, I suggest that within this local framework a strong genetic kinship narrative emerges which surrogates draw upon to distance themselves emotionally from the baby. This distancing, in turn, leads the surrogate to imagine her body as interlinked with the body of the intended mother, creating a shared, embodied intimacy between them. Their relationship humanizes the technologically assisted, contractually arbitrated agreement, transforming it into a gift relationship, which is then incorporated by the surrogate into a heroic narrative. I conclude with some thoughts on the global surrogacy arena from the perspective of this local case and suggest that it may serve as a model for a more ethical surrogacy than that currently practiced within the global framework.

Genetic distancing

The surrogates' navigation of the pregnancy was largely based upon their being completely convinced of the genetic basis of kinship. Whereas Jewish law has historically privileged the womb in establishing kin-ties (Kahn 2000), popular Israeli lay ideas about pregnancy strongly privilege genetics over gestation (Ivry 2009).

Thus, surrogacy participants commonly understood the surrogate to be "hosting" a baby that was not her own because it was not created from her genetic matter.

While the surrogacy law officially regards the surrogate as the "carrying mother," the local popular Hebrew idiom for the surrogate role in the Israeli press and among surrogates themselves constructs the surrogate not as a "mother" but as a "host"; she is referred to as the *pundekait* (innkeeper) and surrogacy is regarded as *pundekaut* (inn-keeping). Surrogates did not want to be viewed in any way as the mother of this child and they reserved the "mother" label for the intended mother, whom they referred to as "the mom" or "the biological mother." They consistently used the inn-keeping idiom as it fit their view of their role as merely hosts of this baby and this family, these weary travelers, on their "journey."

Unlike Indian surrogates, who are "coached" or trained, often unconvincingly, to think about themselves as passive "carriers" of a non-related baby by the clinics arbitrating the agreement (Pande 2011; Harrison 2014; Vora 2014), Israeli surrogates strongly asserted the genetic script "proving" their lack of connection to the baby and consistently downplayed the contribution of their gestation to fetal outcome. Using metaphors such as incubator, oven and hothouse to describe their carrier role, they insisted that they had no difficulty distancing themselves from the baby because they believed that gestation, unlike genetics, has no "bonding" effect. As one surrogate explained:

> I have no connection to this child. It is just like it's called, a literal inn [*pundak*]. I am a guesthouse [*achsania*] for nine months [...] the innkeeper [*pundekait*] only. It is not my egg, and I have no connection to this child.

Surrogates distanced the pregnancy by drawing imaginary lines on their bodies, mapping strictly defined areas with clear boundaries where their personal self ends and their distanced parts begin. One surrogate explained:

> Some [neighbors] said, "Oy vey, she is giving away her children." They just couldn't digest that it wasn't mine ... Nothing, nothing is mine here. It is only theirs [the couple's] ... nothing of him, not my blood. No. It is all theirs ... what was put into me is a whole baby. It is ready. A baby that is formed from the sperm and egg together and was created as a baby and only then inserted into my belly. And then what is attached to me is just in the placenta and the umbilical cord. But nothing else is mine. Nothing, nothing is mine ... And that is why I am telling you, that you don't have feelings [for the baby] like you would expect.

Connecting

Thinking about themselves as distanced genetically and emotionally from the pregnancy led surrogates to imagine their bodies as interlinked with the intended mother's body. This type of imagery was inspired both by the surrogates' desire to distance the pregnancy from their personal "self" and from their understanding of the intended mothers' desire to participate in the pregnancy. It was also facilitated by their frequent communication in person and by phone. As they distanced the pregnancy, surrogates began to develop a sense of having detached the belly into a space that they experienced as disconnected from their body. As one surrogate said of her belly: "[It] wasn't even part of my body … it isn't connected to me … psychologically, it isn't mine, it doesn't connect." Other women expressed this sense of spatial disconnection by saying, "It was as if the pregnancy moved alongside me," or outlining with hand motions directed to the belly area, "I am divided in three. From here to here is me, from here to here isn't me, from here to here is me."

Often, this sense of having detached the belly from their bodies was accompanied by the notion that their intended mother was somehow virtually carrying the belly and pregnancy close to her own body, in a type of shared, disembodied space between them. As one surrogate told me at a surrogacy gathering where her intended mother was also present, "It is like my belly isn't here [nods toward belly with her head]. It is like for this period that my belly is there, with her" [nodding her head to where her intended mother stood, a few yards away].

Whereas surrogates were focused upon disembodying the pregnancy, most of the intended mothers were intent upon becoming as involved in the pregnancy as possible. Some women constituted their ability to have children created from their own eggs and carried by a surrogate as filling out a body image that they had considered defective, disabled, and not "whole" because of their missing reproductive capacity (Teman 2009; 2010a). An intended mother who had lost her womb to cancer recounted her surprise that her husband's family had accepted her so readily "despite what I represent. Because I represent an empty place. Because I have no womb, no potential to give him children."

In contrast, when she spoke about the frozen embryos she had secured before her hysterectomy, she gestured outward with her hands as though encompassing a rounded belly and said: "From the moment that I knew that I had the embryos, I felt like they were right here [gesturing outwards from her belly]. It was as though there was already a pregnancy." Her surrogate, in turn, was conceptualized as the material site of her extension: "I see her as the part of me that is missing. She is my uterus."

This shared imaginary of surrogates and intended mothers that the pregnancy could exist in a space detached from the surrogate's body and attached to the intended mother's embodied space led to interactions between them concerning the sharing and shifting of the pregnant body (Teman 2009). Surrogates would communicate any and all bodily sensations to their intended mothers, both as a distancing technique and in order to defer them onto their counterpart. Surrogates verbally shared everything from nausea and vomiting to cramping, delineating boundaries between what they deemed their personal body and bodily occurrences they deemed "not me." This encouraged their counterpart to identify with the pregnancy, as one intended mother conveyed:

She passed everything she felt on to me. She didn't want to feel it. Not the pregnancy, not the nausea, not the vomiting … She would call right away and transfer them to me ... And she gave me the feeling and the sensation that "it is you – it is you!" ... I felt pregnant. I felt everything that she felt. On the same day that her stomach hurt, my stomach hurt ... Now she, even when she had even the smallest [bout with] nausea, she would call me and I would feel it. I would say to her, "you know what, I feel like it is me".

Identification and intimacy

Body-centered communication between the two women opened up a space for a shared intimacy that was often described as a closeness incomparable to any other intimate relationship, an intimacy they had never shared before with another person (see also Berend 2012 on intimacy in US surrogacy relationships). Surrogates and intended mothers alike tried to fit the relationship into a known category: they compared their relationship to that of sisters, mother and daughter, or best friends. Some described how they seemed to look alike, or had been mistaken for twins. They would joke that they were like lesbian lovers or that they were married to one another during surrogacy, always noting that their unique relationship called for its own category.

At the height of the intended mother's identification with the surrogate, some described instances of telepathy between them. Surrogates reported how their intended mothers would call them and seemingly "know" that the baby inside her had just kicked, or that she was feeling cramps in the left side. One intended mother told me that she had so identified with her surrogate that she intuitively knew when her surrogate's labor began and showed up to wait for her under her house before her surrogate even called to let her know it was time to leave for the hospital.

Surrogates and intended mothers also discussed their intimacy in terms of being merged into one body. Intended mothers described feeling as if they and their surrogate were "two halves of one stomach that unifies us" or unified with their surrogate as "one mind," "one soul," or "one blood stream." The most popular terminology for describing this merging was, as one intended mother put it, "We are one body together that is pregnant." Surrogates also spoke of their bodily connection with their intended mother in terms of sharing the body, in such quotes as "she is me and I am her. We are one body" and "my body is her body now and that is natural."

The women described instances of blurred boundaries and substituting for one another. In six cases, intended mothers told me that they had gained between five and 15 kilograms during the surrogate's pregnancy while their surrogate had gained a minimal amount of weight. Surrogates often noted during post-birth interviews that their bodies had not produced milk, while in two cases intended mothers spontaneously secreted milk after seeing their newborns. One intended mother even reported performing an intuitive couvade-like birth simultaneous to her surrogate's delivery, even though she was not allowed to enter the surgery room:

They gave her (the surrogate) an operation (cesarean section) and I sat outside and I got up and sat down and at one point I fainted. I lost consciousness and collapsed on the floor for eight, nine, ten minutes. And it ends up that exactly at that same moment they extracted them (the twins) from the womb. And everyone said to me, "here you gave birth to them just now." And at that very second I hadn't known what was going on inside and she had gone in already at seven thirty … They elevated my legs and extracted our fetuses; I mean they took our babies out, when I was still on the floor.

The delivery was often described as the height of the women's intimacy; most surrogates encouraged their intended mothers to stand close to them and hold their hand. One surrogate told how she squeezed her intended mother's hand with each contraction so tightly that she left a mark on it, and another surrogate said that as the twins she birthed were being extracted in a cesarean operation, she was more focused on trying to calm her intended mother, who stood next to her shaking, than on what was being done to her body. Many times, this participation made the intended mother feel that she had been central to the delivery: "She told me that without me she couldn't have done it. She said that I helped her give birth."

The identification and intimacy between surrogates and intended mothers existed, however, within carefully drawn boundaries. For surrogates it was always clear that the boundaries of their personal self within the body were complete, bounded and unquestioned. It was only the belly, the experience of pregnancy and their caring sentiments that were "shared" with their intended mother, and there were "red lines" designating the personal self that should not be crossed (Teman 2010a). For intended mothers, on the other hand, the boundaries of the surrogate's offering were not always clear, and the blurred boundaries of their identification and intimacy gave way in some instances to attempts by intended mothers to completely encompass, append and overtake the surrogate's entirety. In such cases, over-identification led to estrangement, and to the surrogate feeling "invaded" and "suffocated" (see Teman 2010a).

At the other extreme, an intended mother's complete lack of participation in the pregnancy, disinterest and emotional distance could leave the surrogate equally dissatisfied. The intended mothers did not necessarily have to append the disembodied belly through pseudo-pregnant embodiment, but surrogates expected them to show an active interest in the pregnancy, accompany them to medical events, interact with them on a routine basis and be their "partner" in the pregnancy. A shared intimacy was expected, and in cases when the intended mother was hesitant or refused to participate in a shared "holding" of the pregnancy, surrogates believed they had more difficulty carrying the disconnected pregnancy without her support. One surrogate, who lamented her intended mother's disinterest in her and in the pregnancy, explained her early term birth as a surrogate – after carrying her own five children full term – as a result of this lack of intimacy: "She didn't help me hold it! And it fell!"

Her words reveal that the surrogate's ability to maintain her disconnections from the pregnancy is partially dependent upon her ability to maintain connections with the intended mother: the surrogate feels she cannot disembody the pregnancy and distance the fetus without the intended mother's reciprocal containment and support. For surrogates, the disembodiment of the pregnancy could only be maintained when the disconnected belly was "held" through the relationship and reciprocally "carried" by the intended mother in a shared "holding" created through intimacy and identification.

Gift and reciprocity

Hand in hand with these expectations of intimacy, surrogates began to perceive their relationship with the intended mother as a "gift relationship" rather than a "business agreement" (Teman 2010a). As one surrogate said: "It begins with the money but it does not end with the money." Surrogates viewed their role as giving more than just a baby through a formal, contractual agreement; they gave another woman their caring, their friendship and the chance to participate in the pregnancy and in this period of "transition to motherhood." Many of the surrogates expressed their commitment to making this couple into parents by saying things like "If I won the lottery tomorrow I would do it for free." Surrogates also began to expect reciprocation beyond the money they received; the reciprocation they expected was in meaningful acknowledgement and recognition by the couple of the enormity of what she had given (Teman 2010a).

While the popular concern is that surrogates may feel traumatized over relinquishing the baby, what emerges from my findings is that surrogates were emotionally fragile after the birth in cases of abrupt separation from the intended mother's companionship rather than because of separation from the newborn. Surrogates had become accustomed to being the focus of much attention throughout the pregnancy. They were the intermediary between the intended parents and the baby, at the center of the whole process. Returning home to their former lives was difficult, as was the reality of knowing that the intended mother was busy with her baby now and no longer had time or the vested interest to be in constant touch with her. Surrogates expressed nervousness towards the end of the pregnancy that they would lose the relationship with the intended mother; after the delivery they would look for signs that they were still important to her even after the contract had ended.

This is where things became delicate: if the intended parents, the intended mother especially, failed to acknowledge the surrogate's contribution as a heartfelt gift rather than a cold contractual exchange, the surrogate emerged regretful and disappointed from the process. If the intended mother cut off all contact immediately after the birth or began to view the surrogate with suspicion, surrogates experienced a profound sense of betrayal. And if the surrogate was reminded by defensive intended parents about the rules of the contract or of the money they had paid her for carrying the baby, it was often interpreted as a very hurtful insult, disrespectful of the enormous amount of "emotional labor" (Hochschild 2003) she had invested in their relationship. As one such surrogate lamented: "I gave this couple my soul and they tricked and betrayed me."

Yet if the surrogate's contribution was reciprocated by meaningful acknowledgement in the form of an emotional "thank you" letter, a heartfelt verbal testimony by the intended parents, or a significant and meaningful gift to the surrogate or to her children expressing acknowledgement of the magnitude of her contribution, the surrogate would feel validated, proud, and empowered by the entire experience (Teman 2010a). An affecting acknowledgement such as one posted on a public surrogacy internet forum or on Facebook for all to see, or one read in front of guests at a birth celebration for the newborn, could make a surrogate feel like everything she had done was worthwhile. Such meaningful acknowledgement could be as simple as an intended mother repeatedly telling her surrogate how indebted she is to her, like one intended mother who said:

> There is something that I always tell her, the surrogate. I say, "My mother gave me life the first time, when she gave birth to me. You gave me life the second time, when you gave birth to my son."

Surrogates who received meaningful acknowledgement would recall their surrogacy experience as the most significant thing they had ever done in their lives. In these accounts, the moment of relinquishment, when they saw their intended mother hold the baby in her arms or saw the intended father's face when he first saw the baby, was the surrogate's proudest and happiest moment. These surrogates would speak of their bond with the intended mother nostalgically, like one speaks of one's comrade in arms or best friend from high school, even if they had not seen the intended mother or spoken to her for several years. In such cases, contact often dropped off gradually during the first few months or years following the birth, but this was not interpreted as an insult because acknowledgement had already been secured (Teman 2010a).

Surrogates who received acknowledgement constructed a heroic narrative of their surrogacy experience, which they relayed with a sense of great pride during our interviews and continued to relay years later. They spoke of themselves as angels or messengers of God. They believed they had done what God, nature, technology and even the best physicians could not do – they gave this couple a baby, and even more significant in Israel's highly familial society, they made this other woman into a mother. These surrogates described the few weeks after delivering the child as feeling a "high" from realizing the magnitude of their actions. As one surrogate who gave birth to twins put it: "No one knows what it is to give, to give life to someone else. I mean, it is like donating your organs while you are still alive."

Conclusion

The case of local, national surrogacy in Israel as discussed in this chapter brings up several notions that might be viewed as a model for a more ethical surrogacy than that which we are currently witnessing in the world. First, because the Israeli surrogates are so convinced by the genetic script of kinship, they truly believe from the outset that the baby is not their own. It is this understanding that enables them to separate emotionally from the baby and from their entitlement to the label of "mother" to this child. Contrast this to the data emergent from the Indian context, where the surrogates seem to be far less convinced of the genetic script. While clinics attempt to persuade them of the "it's not your egg" logic, even leading some Indian surrogates interviewed in Western media to repeat this genetic logic to reporters, it seems that their words only loosely veil much stronger indigenous cultural understandings of pregnancy, privileging gestational kin-ties over genetics.

When clinics try to "train" Indian surrogates to think with the genetic script, it can be viewed as a cruel practice; their basic conceptual framework for thinking about pregnancy is being "discursively colonized" (Bailey 2011) by market interests. Harrison (2014) suggests that Indian surrogates display agency in their resistance to the genetic script. Pande's (2011) interviewees emphasized the contribution of their own "sweat," "blood" and gestational effort over the couple's genetics, while Hochschild (2011) interviewed a surrogate who claimed she was the baby's "real mother." Some Indian surrogates even report bonding with the baby they bore (Rudrappa 2012); I never heard an Israeli surrogate express even a remote sense of bonding with the baby, likely because they were so culturally convinced that this was not their child.

Second, the Israeli data establishes that when parties are close in proximity and share a common spoken language and cultural knowledge, it can open up a space for sharing an intimacy that humanizes the process. The fact that the Israeli women could and did meet frequently and that nearly all of the intended mothers accompanied the surrogate to all medical appointments and were consistently in touch with her put their relationship at the center of the process. It "warmed up" the technologically facilitated, contract-arbitrated procedure (Roberts 1998) and gave the surrogate the feeling that the intended mother was "holding" the pregnancy with her. The intended mother's constant presence supported the surrogates' distancing efforts by enabling surrogates to renounce their potential entitlement to the social label of "mother" of this child by clearly signifying another candidate to whom they assigned that label. The women's relationship also created the basis for the gift logic of reciprocal ties to supercede the contractual agreement.

The Indian data again emerges in sharp contrast because surrogates and couples rarely meet. Often it is the clinic that prevents them from meeting, while in other cases they may meet once or more, but their relationship is not able to grow because of the language barrier and because of deep stereotypes that the foreign couples may hold of their Indian surrogate (Harrison 2014). Pande (2011) found that Indian surrogates do desire a relationship with the intended mother, and that some even imagine or convince themselves of the existence of such a relationship, but that it remains imaginary. Emotional support is garnered from "sisterhood" with other surrogates (Rudrappa 2012), rather than from a relationship with the couple. The "gift" remains merely rhetoric, as there is no basis for reciprocal relations. In the absence of a relationship between the two sides of the agreement, surrogacy remains a cold, unequal, contractual commodity exchange.

Third, the Israeli case, in stark contrast to the global case, shows that when surrogacy is strictly regulated there is far less of a chance for legal entanglements to occur. Many of the horror stories we hear today through the media stem from lack of regulation. Protections are set out in the contract in order to ensure the future of the newborn. The baby is entitled to Israeli citizenship upon birth, unlike babies born of some cross-national arrangements in which parents must prove a genetic link to the baby through a DNA test before the baby is granted citizenship in the parents' home country. This prevents situations such as those emerging out of India of newborns that no nation will grant citizenship to.[3] Moreover, intended parents must take custody of the newborn under penalty of law, and cannot refuse to accept a special needs baby. If they are unable to take custody for some outstanding reason, guardians are written into the contract who will take custody in their stead. This prevents situations such as the recent case in Thailand when intended parents refused to accept a baby born to them through surrogacy who had Down Syndrome, and the surrogate was left to raise him.

The screening of all candidates for entering into surrogacy contracts also prevents many complications. In Israel all intended parents undergo criminal background checks in order to prevent cases such as the recent case in Thailand of an intended father who was revealed post-surrogacy to be a convicted pedophile (Whittaker, this volume). The number of surrogacy contracts a couple can enter into is also strictly limited, preventing cases such as the recent headlining case in Thailand of a Japanese man fathering fourteen children through Thai surrogacy services (ibid).

Surrogates in Israel are tested, pre-contract, for psychological and physical health so as to prevent any risk to her health or the baby's health because of the process; if anything, the surrogacy committee is too restrictive in its criteria for who can become a surrogate and too paternalistic towards intended parents, but the restrictions prevent outcomes seen in cross-border surrogacy. A potential Israeli surrogate can be disqualified for already having given birth to four babies, for having been a surrogate twice before or having given birth twice by cesarean; she cannot have had certain types of plastic surgery in the past, had gestational diabetes or early term births, or taken anti-depressants (Teman 2010b). On the other hand, contracting couples are not suddenly surprised to learn medical information about their surrogate after having already attempted multiple embryo transfers, as is frequently reported in the news media regarding unregulated contexts such as Georgia, Mexico and elsewhere.

Finally, cases such as those reported from India of surrogates not receiving the funds promised or not understanding the details of the contract (Deomampo 2013) are prevented in Israel because the committee requires the couple to deposit all funding up front with an attorney; the surrogate is also interviewed by the committee before contract approval and it "tests" her on the contract details to ensure she is fully aware of what she is signing (Teman 2010a). Elsewhere (Teman 2010b), I have critiqued this law for its restrictiveness and argued that legislators passed it so as to ensure that local surrogacy will only produce Jewish-Israeli citizens to heteronormative, nuclear families. Yet it is in light of what goes on in the global arena that one can see that the Israeli surrogacy law has contributed to a humanization of surrogacy and can serve as a model for what can make surrogacy relatively more ethical.

Notes

1 In 2013 the committee grudgingly began to allow married surrogates, three years after the chief rabbinical authority had ruled it halakhically permissible. The committee's decision to allow married surrogates came primarily in light of increasing demand for surrogacy and the small pool of unmarried candidates volunteering to become surrogates.
2 This article is based upon this ethnographic study of surrogacy arrangements in Israel. The study encompassed multiple sites and methods (see Teman 2010a for full details), including qualitative interviews with 26 gestational surrogates and 35 intended mothers involved in gestational surrogacy arrangements, some of whom were repeatedly interviewed throughout the surrogacy process.
3 In such arrangements, if the baby is revealed to be the surrogate's genetic offspring because of a lapse in the fertilization process, legal hurdles between Indian and foreign law often prevent the intended parents taking the baby out of India and into their home country even if the surrogate agrees.

References

Bailey, Alison. 2011. Reconceiving surrogacy: Toward a reproductive justice account of Indian surrogacy. *Hypatia* 26(4):715–741.
Berend, Zsuzsa. 2012. The Romance of Surrogacy. *Sociological Forum* 27(4):913–936.
Deomampo, Daisy. 2013. Transnational surrogacy in India: Interrogating power and women's agency. *Frontiers: A Journal of Women Studies* 34(3):167–188.
Donath, Orna. 2010. Pro-natalism and its 'Cracks': Narratives of Reproduction and Childfree Lifestyles in Israel. *Israeli Sociology* 11(2):417–439.
Harrison, Laura. 2014. "I am the baby's real mother": Reproductive tourism, race, and the transnational construction of kinship. *Women's Studies International Forum* 47:145–156.
Hochschild, Arlie Russell. 2003. *The managed heart: Commercialization of human feeling, with a new afterword*. Berkeley, CA: University of California Press.
Hochschild, Arlie Russell. 2011. Childbirth at the global crossroads. In Anita Ilta Garey, Karen V. Hansen (eds), *At the heart of work and family: Engaging the ideas of Arlie Hochschild*, pp. 262–269. New Brunswick, NJ: Rutgers University Press.
Ivry, Tsipy. 2009. *Embodying culture: pregnancy in Japan and Israel*. New Brunswick, NJ: Rutgers University Press.
Kahn, Susan Martha. 2000. *Reproducing Jews: A Cultural Account of Assisted Conception in Israel*. Durham, NC: Duke University Press.
Pande, Amrita. 2011. Transnational commercial surrogacy in India: gifts for global sisters? *Reproductive Biomedicine Online* 23(5):618–625.
Roberts, Elizabeth F.S. 1998. "Native" Narratives of Connectedness: Surrogate Motherhood and Technology. In Robbie Davis-Floyd and Joseph Dumit (eds), *Cyborg Babies: From Techno-Sex to Techno-Tots*, pp. 193–211. New York, NY: Routledge.
Rudrappa, Sharmila. 2012. India's reproductive assembly line. *Contexts* 11(2):22–27.
Teman, Elly. 2009. Embodying Surrogate Motherhood: Pregnancy as a Dyadic Body Project. *Body and Society* 15(3):47–57.
Teman, Elly. 2010a. *Birthing a Mother: The Surrogate Body and the Pregnant Self*. Berkeley, CA: University of California Press.

Teman, Elly. 2010b. The Last Outpost of the Nuclear Family: A Cultural Critique of Israeli Surrogacy Policy. In D. Birenbaum-Carmeli and Y. Carmeli (eds), *Kin, Gene, Community: Reproductive Technology among Jewish Israelis*, pp. 107–126. Oxford, UK: Berghahn Books.

Vora, Kalindi. 2014. Experimental sociality and gestational surrogacy in the Indian ART clinic. *Ethnos* 79(1):63–83.

14 From manufacturing clothes to manufacturing babies

Economic precarity and labor options among surrogate mothers in Bangalore, India

Sharmila Rudrappa

Introduction

"*Aiyo akka*, we garment workers ... our lives are hell. And our worlds are destroyed," declared Lalitha dramatically. It was the end of my first field visit to the southern Indian city of Bangalore to research surrogacy. I had not expected to study the garment industry, but many of the surrogate mothers I met were formerly garment workers, or their mothers had worked in garment factories. In our conversations the women constantly contrasted their employment as surrogate mothers to their work in garment factories. I had not expected it when I first began studying transnational surrogacy, but tracing the paths of post-industrial cross-border reproductive care, I found myself at the doorstep of industrial garment work. Many of the Bangalore surrogate mothers I met moved in and out of sweatshops manufacturing garments for a global market to reproductive assembly lines to "manufacture" babies.

While there are accounts of Indian women's experiences *as* surrogate mothers (Pande 2010, 2011; Deomampo 2013a, 2013b) there is almost nothing on *why* women choose surrogacy as a wage option. Working from the premise that prior work experiences shape the ways individuals choose and feel about current employment, I maintain that in order to understand surrogate mothers, we need to appreciate their personal working histories. Thus, the two interrelated questions I explore in this chapter are as follows: first, what are the surrogate mothers' prior working histories, and how might these past engagements partially explain why they become surrogate mothers, and their feelings about surrogacy? Many women contrasted labor processes in garment sweatshops and surrogacy to explain *why* they became surrogate mothers. In spite of the deep, bodily interventions entailed in surrogacy, many of the surrogate mothers posited that surrogacy empowered them. Taking my cue from the surrogate mothers I met with, I look at garment factories to understand why they deemed surrogacy a viable labor option.

This chapter is organized in the following manner: following this introduction I describe my methods. Next, I explain how Bangalore's surrogate mothers are recruited from garment factories. Because so many of the women's lives follow similar trajectories, for narrative purposes, I focus primarily on one surrogate mother I call Indirani. Indirani, a former garment worker, was 30 years old when I met her, and was pregnant with twins for a Tamil couple who lived in the United States. Through detailing Indirani's life story I map the garment industry–surrogacy nexus in Bangalore. I then conclude with thoughts on why women choose surrogacy as work, and find such work life affirming. These structures of feelings – of helplessness, self-worth, agency, and empowerment through surrogacy – do not arise out of thin air, but have a social context. This context, I argue, as do the surrogate mothers, is the decreasing value of Third World working-class women's labor in neoliberal economies. Growing precariousness in sweatshops, which results in the evisceration of working-class families in Bangalore, I argue, leads these women to find work in reproductive assembly lines as life-affirming developments.

Methods

This chapter is based on my fieldwork in Bangalore, southern India, begun as a participant observer in an infertility clinic (summer 2008 and 2009), which led to ethnographic research among surrogate mothers in the city. In March 2011 I spent two weeks at a surrogacy dormitory that I call Creative Options for Women, COTW. I learned that many of the ten residents there were formerly garment workers. Over 2011 I re-interviewed the ten mothers I had met in COTW; they had all delivered their babies and left the dormitory's premises. Through these ten women I met and interviewed 60 others, many of whom had already surrogated, or were pregnant. By December 2011 I had interviewed 70 surrogate mothers, and conducted focus groups with 22 garment workers (who were not surrogate mothers). I also interviewed 31 egg donors.

Choosing ideal women for surrogacy

"If you asked me two years ago whether I'd have a baby and give it away for money, I wouldn't just laugh at you, I would be so insulted I might hit you in the face," said Indirani, in apparent disbelief that she had changed so much in two years. She had delivered twins a month earlier for a Tamil couple who lived in the United States, for which she had received US $4,000. Typical of the 70 surrogate mothers I met in Bangalore, 30-year-old Indirani and her husband were not poor, but they struggled to make meet ends meet. Married at 18, Indirani had a son and a daughter, both of whom were under ten years of age. Both children attended a private school because Indirani and her husband wanted their children to have greater economic stability than either of them had in their lives. Indirani earned US $100 to $110 per month as a garment worker, and her husband drove a rented auto-rickshaw to earn money. The daily rental and gasoline costs for the vehicle cut significantly into the household income, so the couple borrowed money to purchase an auto-rickshaw of their own. But always late on paying loan installments, they realized they were in a financial crisis. When a friend at the garment factory she worked at suggested that she sell her eggs for approximately US $500, Indirani jumped at the opportunity. Next, she tried surrogacy and got pregnant at the first attempt with twins.

A commonplace understanding is that women who are desperately poor become surrogate mothers. Yet, my research shows that this is not true. Most of the women I met in Bangalore are like Indirani; they come from dominant castes, from solidly working-class families, and live in multi-generational households with multiple adults pooling their resources to make ends meet. Almost all the mothers I met wanted private schooling for their children. They often incurred debts in order to make investments to stabilize their familial economic status, provide better housing, or because of an illness in the family. And many were garment workers, because the city's garment industry, which produced for national and international markets, was the largest contingent employer for working-class women.

Considered ideal candidates for surrogacy, as I subsequently explain, agencies actively sought persons like Indirani in women-centric spaces such as garment factories. Surrogacy agencies do *not* recruit poverty-stricken women because they may be malnourished, their health compromised through years of living in poverty. They may have poor dental health. And because they lack permanent housing and adequate supplies of potable water, they may not have the prerequisite ideals of bodily hygiene apparent in clean clothing, sandals on their feet, hair that is neatly oiled, combed, and coiffed. Recruiters prefer women who come from solid working-class backgrounds and live in permanent housing, have access to water to bathe daily and wash their clothes, and can afford to eat regular, healthy meals. Such women are not only in better health, but also, they present well to clients.

However, it is not enough for surrogacy agencies to bring women to the dormitory and expect them to engage in reproductive work. Like other firms, in order to create surplus value, surrogacy agencies need to solicit labor effort from their workers, either by using subtle means of coercion or by mobilizing workers' consent (Bowles and Gintis 1990). Highly dependent on women to get pregnant and deliver babies for clients, surrogacy agencies must have a disciplined workforce. The women must be prepared to receive high dosages of synthetic hormones and agree to invasive medical procedures including caesarean deliveries. And crucially, the surrogate mothers are screened for, and coached against, engaging in "post-contractual opportunistic behavior" (Galbraith, McLachlan, and Swales 2005), that is, making demands on intended parents during their pregnancies and after the babies are born. The latter is achieved partially because of the vast differences between surrogate mothers and the intended parents; geographical distance, racial hierarchies, cultural incommensurability, and class differences create close to insurmountable barriers between the two. In addition, surrogate agencies minimize contact between workers and clients; for example, clients are not allowed to meet with mothers without agency supervision. Agency staff mediate translations between English and whatever languages the Indian women may speak. And, finally, staff must be apprised of all gifts intended parents give to surrogate mothers. Many intended parent interviewees said they were not allowed to communicate with the surrogate mothers without prior permission from the agency.

The challenge for agencies, however, is not the mothers' post-contractual opportunistic behavior; instead, the most capital-intensive task lies in disciplining the mothers on the reproductive factory shop-floor. In her ethnography of surrogate mothers in Anand, Gujarat Amrita Pande (2010) describes how women are shaped into what she terms "mother workers". They are similar to factory workers but are simultaneously caring mothers who are produced through counseling, contractual agreements that enforce them to surrender babies, and through installing them for months on end – separate from their own social worlds – in surrogacy dormitories with other women like them. Through coordinating activities according to schedules over the course of the day, week, and months in the dormitories, industrial discipline is inculcated in the women, which the infertility clinic harnesses to accumulate surplus value.

While Pande (2010) focuses on the processes that engender mothers' acquiescence after they have signed on to become surrogate mothers, I argue that women's consent *prior* to even entering the labor contract is crucial. Surrogacy agencies need women who are accustomed to industrial discipline, rather than someone who learns about compliance and contracts on the job. Thus, recruitment of ideal candidates is an important task for surrogacy agencies. COTW, the surrogacy agency that recruited most of the mothers I interviewed, is located in the heart of one of Bangalore's garment neighborhoods; agents recruit from amongst the women who live in the vicinity, most of whom are garment workers.[1] But this still begs the question: why do garment workers like Indirani believe that surrogacy is a good labor option? To understand why necessarily leads me back to the doorstep of the garment industry in Bangalore.

Garment production in India

Like most other developing countries, India's economy is dominated by textile and garment production, which is estimated to account for 26% of the manufacturing output (Gereffi and Guler 2010).[2] In 1960–1961, garment exports were valued at US $2 million; by 1999–2000, garment exports had grown to US $4.765 billion (Chowdhury 2005). Growth in exports has led to a rise in wages, but garment workers are the worst paid industrial workers in India (Barrientos, Mathur, and Sood 2010). Almost 93% of the garment workers are in the unorganized sector, which means that they are not entitled to state-regulated working conditions and social security benefits.

Bangalore, the capital of Karnataka, is the largest garment producer for the state, with the most feminized workforce in all of India. Eighty-four per cent of garment workers are women, and 80% of them are below 30 years of age (Tewari 2010). A vast majority of these workers have completed middle school, and 60% belong to dominant castes (Pani and Singh n.d.: 19–35). The women I interviewed earned between US $50 to $100 every month. A few of the women, who had worked for over 15 years, earned close to $150 per month.

Work in Bangalore's garment factories

Prior to its rise in global prominence as the center of outsourced information technology work from various parts of the world, textiles dominated Bangalore's industry from 1900 to 1950 (Srinivas 2001). From World War II, however, Bangalore's industrial landscape began to change. Srinivas (2001) explains that high-tech, state-sponsored industries were established in the city in the early 1950s; by the 1960s, national research centers such as the Indian Space Research Organization and the Central Power Research Institute were also inaugurated in the city. These capital-intensive, state-sponsored public sector initiatives were accompanied by the development of private subsidiary factories that produced machine parts, tools, and plastic goods (Srinivas 2001).

A large part of this private growth was abetted by the government's small-scale industries' policy that provided subsidies for small, privately owned units. For example, in 1966, through land acquisitions acts, the Karnataka Industrial Areas Development Board established the Peenya industrial district on the outskirts of the city to cater to the needs of small-scale industries. Currently, almost 70% of the city's garment units are located in this industrial belt that runs from the west of the city down to its southern end (Pani and Singh n.d.). Today, Bangalore's garment industry comprises numerous small and large firms, with global clients such as Nike, Adidas, GAP, Abercrombie and Fitch, Levi's, H&M, and Columbia.[3]

Thus, paralleling its growth as a high-tech city, for which it is renowned, Bangalore has witnessed the rapid expansion of low-tech factories including garment production. Amongst Bangalore's 8.5 million denizens, just as ubiquitous as the male software engineer is the female garment worker, rushing every morning, lunch bag in hand, to board the bus to get to a sweatshop. Research shows that Bangalore's female garment workers put in over 16 hours of work a day at the factory and at home. Their most time-consuming chores outside the factory are laundry, cooking, childcare, and commuting to work (Tewari 2010).

In my first fieldwork trip to Bangalore in March 2011, I learned that many of the ten surrogate mothers in COTW's dormitory were garment workers. So I got together with 15 garment workers in one of their homes one evening to talk about their work lives. Many of them began with the same description: "*Bhari* heat *akka. Bhari heat-u.*" I assumed they were telling me that ventilation was poor and women felt uncomfortably hot. "Don't you have water bottles?" I asked. Some women nodded, but others said they did not drink water at work because they would then want to urinate and take more restroom breaks. Sita, who had hosted the focus group, explained that "*heat-u*" was a reference to the body's tendency to "heat up", manifested in urinary tract infections (UTIs). The women explained that they attracted the attention of the male supervisors when they did not meet production quotas. The women did not want this attention because these men castigated them in sexual terms and sometimes groped them to humiliate them in front of their co-workers. To avoid such sexual degradation the women worked continuously without taking breaks. Most of them used the restrooms only during the midday 45-minute lunch break, and upon completion of work around 6:00pm.

I have no first-hand data on workers' health, but research in Dhaka, Bangladesh shows that garment workers suffered from headaches, chest pain, ear and eye pain, general anemia, gastritis, nausea, cough, cold and other forms of respiratory difficulties, UTIs, and reproductive health problems. Nearly 18% of the Dhaka women surveyed had suffered from UTIs the previous month. Of these, 40% of the women said they had UTIs for almost an entire month. The Dhaka workers said they put in 12-hour days at work, and there was no provision for paid leave. The average length of a garment worker's working life was four years (Majumdar 2003).

The 15 garment workers I met with in Sita's house said that the production quotas were set at such high levels that they were unable to meet them in spite of not taking breaks. So they stayed after work hours to finish up, but did not receive overtime wages. Supervisors claimed the women had wasted time during the workday, and did not deserve overtime pay. When paychecks did not reflect their overtime work, husbands and in-laws wondered whether the women were really at the factory, or whether they were having an extramarital affair. As a result women reported that they felt degraded at work by their supervisors and at home by castigating family members.

In her study of maquiladoras, Melissa Wright (2006) explains that by creating value on the shop-floor, working-class women depreciate in value themselves. The key to this conversion, Wright says, lies in the work process. Because of the long work hours and the repetitive work in sweatshops, the workers' health deteriorates. Over time they are unable to sustain their productivity and are fired. They become disposable byproducts of the industrial process who are then replaced by new workers. Employers posit that women are replaced frequently in factories because their biological destinies as mothers and devotion to family dominate their lives. Thus, the high turnover among women workers is posited as *their* choice rather than as caused by bad jobs.

Just as Wright (2006) describes, in Bangalore's garment factories women constantly shift from being valuable workers to becoming waste. When a woman is healthy she produces value for the firm; but when she is sick, has familial obligations, or is simply exhausted because of factory labor, she loses her value as a worker. She is replaced. Upon recovering her health or managing family chores effectively, she cycles back into garment factories again, this time having regained her value for the industrial process. The women I interviewed strive against the conditions in factories and at home that leave them exhausted. With few exceptions, their contingent employment in garment factories is over by their mid-30s.

These sorts of labor processes, I maintain, shape women's subjectivities regarding wage work. Contingent work, fragile ties between employer and employee, exhaustion on the shop-floor, and finally, the nature of the product itself – that is, making garments versus making babies – had two effects. First, these processes habituated garment workers to the industrial discipline that was required in surrogacy. And second, workers themselves compared garment work to surrogacy, and posited the latter as ideal work. In the following section I expand on these four aspects of industrial and post-industrial production to illuminate why women felt that surrogacy was life affirming.

The instability of work

Garment production is highly dependent on contracts received from global retailers. When Bangalore factories receive contracts, they need large numbers of workers to meet production quotas on schedule; at other times, when work-orders are small or they have not received contracts, they do not need workers on the payroll. For the women workers, then, there are periods when workloads are extraordinarily heavy, followed by periods when there is no work at all because they are downsized. As a result, working conditions and wages are erratic. They are either overworked and receive wages, or months go by before they receive a paycheck. To deal with such contingency, they become dependent on high-interest rate loans. They borrow when they are downsized, sick, and unable to work, and otherwise need funds to cover daily living expenses. Their debts balloon out of control rapidly. Upon finding employment again, a sizeable part of their paychecks go toward servicing their debts taken from usurious moneylenders.

Under these conditions of economic instability and debt dependence, selling their ova and surrogacy at COTW are appealing. The women believed they could earn up to US $4,000 from a single pregnancy to pay off their loans, and build a savings account for times of economic need.

Fragile ties

The garment workers' families' economic instability was exacerbated because they lacked social ties with persons from privileged class positions. The situation was somewhat different for Bangalore's women of the same class background, but employed in non-industrial jobs. For example, domestic workers such as maids, house cleaners, and nannies relied on their employers for short-term loans. The nature of domestic work was such that employers and employees formed exploitative and hierarchical but *enduring* social bonds. Employees could petition their employers to provide interest-free loans, or cash gifts in case children fell sick or husbands lost jobs. Or, some employers paid for private schooling for the maids' children. Though domestic workers often made lower monthly wages than garment workers, their employment was stable, and they could rely on their employers' charity, attended by all the power inequalities that such charity entailed. Thus, domestic workers were less amenable to signing on as surrogate mothers because of job stability and because their employers gave them interest-free loans or cash gifts. In the garment industry, on the other hand, employers and employees lacked ties of allegiance. Contingent work led to contingent social relationships, and garment workers had very few advantageous nodes on their social networks.

Degradation as a garment worker

Surrogate mother Indirani said she felt physically and emotionally exhausted when she worked as a tailor in the factory and then returned to care for her family.

Upon getting pregnant, Indirani relocated to the COTW dormitory and missed her family. She felt isolated among strangers, and worried about whether her mother-in-law was taking care of her children. But soon she began to appreciate dorm life because surrogacy afforded her the luxury of being served by others. Someone else cooked and cleaned for her. She did not have to wake up by 5:00am to prepare meals for her family, pack lunches, drop the children off at the bus stop so they could get to school, and then get to work herself. She had no household obligations, and no one made demands on her time, energy, and emotions. Indirani did not remember a time when she felt so rested and liberated from all responsibilities.

Many mothers told me that initially they felt alone, but as they spent time with surrogate mothers in the dormitory, they recognized they had more in common with each other than with family members, or women friends. Some women told me that they had lost a baby forever but gained sisters for life. "But don't the closed-circuit cameras in the dormitories bother you?" I asked. Many women said they did not register the closed-circuit cameras' presence because surveillance at the dormitory was benign in comparison to the surveillance and punishment meted out on the garment shop-floor, where conversations, taking rest, or going on breaks were all curtailed.

Surrogacy was empowering precisely because of their sensual, sexual, reproductive bodies. If in garment factories they felt degraded because of sexual harassment on the shop-floor, as surrogate mothers they lived in women-only dormitories and relatively free from unwanted sexual attention. Bangalore's reproduction industry, the women expressed, allowed them to be moral workers. They abstained from sex, even with their husbands, and they made babies without engaging in sex. If they were mistreated because of their female bodies on the garment shop-floor, then in surrogacy, it was only through their unique biological capacities as women that they earned US $4,000, gifting extended families with new opportunities, which greatly strengthened their hand in familial decision-making processes, and gave them social status.

Perversely, then, surrogacy afforded them an opportunity to feel rested, make everlasting friendships with other women, and finally, they felt affirmed as *women* in their working and social worlds.

The nature of the product itself

Surrogate mother Indirani contrasted the inherent value in producing babies versus producing garments. She said, "Garments? You wear your shirt a few months and you throw it away. But I make you a baby? You keep that for life." The mothers explained that creating life was incomparable to anything they had accomplished as workers. They added richness to social existence that no other forms of wage labor could generate. By birthing a baby, Indirani said she had fulfilled another woman's desire to be a mother. That woman's infertile marriage, she believed, was stabilized and secured because the couple now had a baby to love together. Moreover, she had contributed to the continuation of patriarchal familial lineage.

Indirani and the mothers I met did *not* misread their exploitation on Bangalore's reproductive assembly lines; nor did they see selling their ova or surrogacy as harmless processes. However, given their options, they believed that Bangalore's reproduction industry afforded them greater control over their emotional, financial, and sexual lives. And finally, babies were meaningful in a way garments were not, and surrogacy was a profoundly creative form of wage employment that allowed women to assert their moral worth.

Concluding thoughts: the myth of dual labor markets and surrogacy as empowerment

Descriptions of late capitalism map a shift from Fordism, dominated by blue-collar jobs, to post-Fordism, with the rise of service jobs and information technologies. From being immersed in the world of material labor, producing shirts, car parts, and such, post-Fordist workers now engage in immaterial labor, where services are produced. Yet, my work on Bangalore shows that not only do industrial and post-industrial workplaces occupy the exact same geographical locales, but also, they employ the exact same people. Bangalore's women transfer their labor from garment production to the reproduction trade, and back to garments again. Insecure conditions in one facet of production create, and sustain, labor markets in others. Fordist and post-Fordist firms inadvertently facilitate each other's existence through fostering specific forms of working conditions for Third World women.

The vagaries of the market and economic risks inherent in garment production are systematically displaced from big, global retailers onto production units that dot various parts of the Third World. These risks, then, are shifted onto individual workers, who take on contingent work, long hours, and hazardous working conditions to make discounted garments that saturate retail outlets. The instability of work on the garment shop-floor in Bangalore is driven by the cycle of global demand, and the less than ideal working conditions are compelled by production deadlines set by global apparel retailers such as Nike and Old Navy.

Paralleling these sorts of developments, the Indian government has pursued structural adjustment policies (SAPs) to enhance free markets and integration into the global economy. SAPs have resulted in an overall growth in GDP, a rise in trade, and an astonishing expansion of high-end consumables. But also, SAPs have resulted in decreased government expenditure on social welfare (Saadatmand, Toma, and Menon 2007). Quality of state-funded schooling has been compromised. Food is costly. Health care is inadequate in public hospitals, and expensive in private hospitals.

Life for garment workers in Bangalore is precarious. Precarious work changes not just the way people work, but also the way they organize their lives (Hewison and Kalleberg 2013: 396). Bangalore's garment workers are not different. They comprehend the social changes occurring around them, and want better opportunities for their children. They invest in their children's education, which translates to higher tuition in private schools. Moreover, because of contingent work in garment sweatshops, workers depend on short-term, high-interest loans.

And finally, sustenance strategies among working-class families in Third World cities such as Bangalore necessitate men and women to optimize their labor potential. Their optimization strategies oblige them to move from industrial production to post-industrial production in order to cope with the precarity of urban life. Under these conditions, Bangalore's reproduction industry offers hope.

While I recognize that the reproduction industry is undoubtedly profit oriented at the expense of surrogate mothers' health (Sarojini and Sharma 2009; Shah 2009; Qadeer 2010), my purpose here is to understand why women *still* sign on as surrogate mothers even when they recognize the risks involved. These sorts of choices, and the conversion of the deep alienation in surrogacy into empowerment, I argue, can only be understood within the context of the Third World women's working lives. Garment work for many women is as Lalitha describes; their lives are hell, and their worlds destroyed. Alternatively, surrogacy becomes a way by which they attempt to create new worlds.

Notes

1 Recruiting agents also have extensive networks among women in their prime fertility who work as maids or are housewives. These women, however, are highly under-represented in Bangalore's reproductive industry. Recruiters' largest success is among garment workers. I argue that this is primarily because the garment industry trains women into industrial discipline. Maids, on the hand, have looser notions of time schedules, hierarchical but closer relationships with employers and their families, and because of that, are able to mobilize gift-like relationships that are hard to engender in garment sweatshops. As a result, they are far less suitable as surrogate mothers than are garment workers.
2 However, garments contribute to only 4% of the gross domestic product.
3 According to www.gokaldas.com (accessed on September 22, 2011).

References

Barrientos Stephanie, M. Mathur, and A. Sood, "Decent Work in Global Production Networks," in *Labour in Global Production Networks in India.* Edited by Anne Posthuma and Dev Nathan, pp. 127–145 (New Delhi: Oxford University Press, 2010).
Bowles Samuel and Herbert Gintis, "Contested Exchange: New Microfoundations for the Political Economy of Capitalism," *Politics and Society*, 18(2):165–222 (1990).
Chowdhury S.R., "Labour Activism and Women in the Unorganized Sector: Garment Export Industry in Bangalore," *Economic and Political Weekly*, 40(22):2,250–2,255 (May 28–June 4, 2005).
Deomampo Daisy, "Gendered Geographies of Reproductive Tourism," *Gender & Society*, 27(4):514–537 (2013a).
Deomampo Daisy, "Transnational Surrogacy in India: Interrogating Power and Women's Agency," *Frontiers: A Journal of Women Studies*, 34(3):167–188 (2013b).
Galbraith Mhairi, Hugh V. McLachlan, and J. Kim Swales, "Commercial Agencies and Surrogate Motherhood: A Transaction Cost Approach," *Health Care Analysis*, 11(25):11–31 (March 2005).
Gereffi Gary and E. Guler, "Global Production Networks and Decent Work in India and China," in Anne Posthuma and Dev Nathan (eds), *Labour in Global Production Networks in India*, pp. 103–126. (New Delhi: Oxford University Press, 2010).

Hewison Kevin and Arne L. Kalleberg, "Precarious Work and Flexibilization in South and Southeast Asia," *American Behavioral Scientist*, 57(4):395–402 (2013).

Majumdar Pratima Paul, *Health Status of the Garment Workers in Bangladesh*. Project Report. Dhaka: Bangladesh Institute of Development Studies (2003).

Pande Amrita, "Commercial Surrogacy in India: Manufacturing a Perfect Mother Worker," *Signs*, 35(4):969–992 (2010).

Pande Amrita, "Transnational Commercial Surrogacy in India: Gifts for Global Sisters?" *Reproductive BioMedicine Online*, 23: 618–625 (2011).

Pani Narendar and Nikky Singh, *The Borders Within: Women, Work, and the Family at the Far End of Globalization* (Bangalore: The National Institute for Advanced Studies, n.d.).

Qadeer Imrana, "The ART of Marketing Babies," *The Indian Journal of Medical Ethics*, VII(4):209–215 (2010).

Saadatmand Yassaman, Michael Toma, and Shyam Menon, "Female Labor Participation in India and Structural Adjustment," *Journal of Global Business Issues*, 1:65–73 (2007).

Sarojini Nadimpally and Aastha Sharma. "The Draft ART (Regulation) Bill: In Whose Interest?" *The Indian Journal of Medical Ethics*, VI(1):36–37 (2009).

Shah Chayanika, "Regulate technology, not lives: A critique of the draft ART (Regulation) bill," *The Indian Journal of Medical Ethics*, VI(1):32–35 (2009).

Srinivas Smriti, *Landscapes of Urban Memory: The Sacred and the Civic in India's High Tech City* (Minneapolis: University of Minnesota Press, 2001).

Tewari Meenu, "Footloose Capital, Intermediation, and the Search for the 'High Road' in Low Wage Industries," in *Labour in Global Production Networks in India*, pp. 146–165 (2010).

Wright Melissa. *Disposable Women and Other Myths of Global Capitalism* (New York: Routledge, 2006).

Index

Page numbers in italic refer to figures. Page numbers in bold refer to tables.